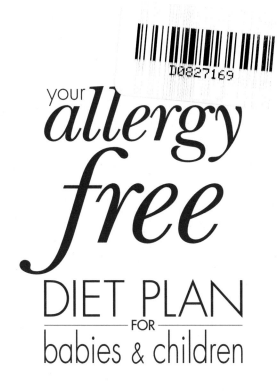

your allergy *free*

DIET PLAN
—— FOR ——
babies & children

carolyn humphries

foulsham
LONDON • NEW YORK • TORONTO • SYDNEY

foulsham

The Publishing House, Bennetts Close,
Cippenham, Slough, Berks, SL1 5AP, England

Additional dietary advice from Tanya Wright, BSc (Hons),
State Registered Dietician, specialist allergy dietician and
adviser to Allergy UK and the Anaphylaxis Campaign.

ISBN 0-572-02891-1

Neither the editors of W. Foulsham & Co. Ltd nor
the author nor the publisher take responsibility for
any possible consequences from any treatment,
procedure, test, exercise, action or application of
medication or preparation by any person reading or
following the information in this book. The
publication of this book does not constitute the
practice of medicine, and this book does not
attempt to replace any diet or instructions from
your doctor. The author and publisher advise the
reader to check with a doctor before administering
any medication or undertaking any course of
treatment or exercise.

Printed in Great Britain by Creative Print and Design (Wales), Ebbw Vale

CONTENTS

INTRODUCTION

Allergies of all kinds are affecting an increasing number of people of all ages, and when they affect the very young, they can be a particular problem. Babies and young children, for example, can't tell you exactly what is wrong, or assess whether a specific food affects them in one way or another. Allergic reactions can be more severe and – of course – we worry about our children and want the very best for them. In addition, adults may well put up with a substitute recipe or food even if they don't particularly like it because they know they can't tolerate the 'real thing' but a child is just as likely to spit it out if it is not what they like.

The information and the recipes in this book are designed specifically to help you produce a healthy, balanced diet for your baby or child, no matter what allergies or intolerances he may have.

Allergic reactions to food show themselves in many different ways. If your baby or child has a frequent upset tummy or constipation, a rash or persistent cough, or is fractious, difficult to handle or simply not thriving as well as he should, it is possible that he may have a food intolerance or allergy. Thankfully, the majority of children grow out of them by the time they go to school; although a few will have a problem for life. For instance, there is growing evidence that some children with autistic spectrum disorders cannot process gluten or milk protein properly. Marked improvements have been noted when these foods have been eliminated from the diet and suitable alternatives substituted.

If you have concerns about your child, the first thing to do is to take him to your doctor for a full medical assessment. Please note that although I have referred to your child as 'him', there is no significance in this. All the advice in this book applies equally to boys and girls. This book is not designed as an alternative to seeking medical advice. It aims to offer a healthy, nutritious and enjoyable diet for children already diagnosed as having a food allergy or intolerance. It starts with the specific problems associated with babies, and how to wean them on to suitable food – this is particularly important if your family has a history of food allergies. It then moves on to catering for an allergic child.

It's hard enough feeding a growing youngster at the best of times but if you have to cut out many of the most popular foods, the job is that much more difficult. With this in mind, I've created versions of most children's favourites, plus some exciting new dishes, to produce varied, balanced, healthy and enjoyable meals.

All the recipes are free of all the **major allergens** (wheat, gluten, dairy products, soya, oats, rye, barley and eggs) but I have added a 'variations' box for those who can tolerate some of the foods that commonly cause allergies. So, for example, if your child can tolerate eggs, the variations table lists the quantity of eggs to be used instead of the egg replacer in the main recipe.

I've included a main course section on fish because, although it is an allergen for some, it is a hugely beneficial source of protein, essential fatty acids, vitamins and minerals for most children. Obviously, if your child can't eat fish, simply ignore that section altogether!

Please note that I have included **minor allergens**, such as citrus fruit and tomatoes, in the recipes, because they will not be a problem for the majority of children. However, wherever these are included, I've given an alternative in the recipe introduction, so you've got the widest range of ideas for great meals for your child every day.

DEALING WITH ALLERGIES AND INTOLERANCES

This chapter looks at the differences between an allergy and an intolerance, and at the specific problems caused by the most common ones. It gives details as to where common allergens hide in processed foods and the best ways to avoid them.

ALLERGY OR INTOLERANCE?

It is a common assumption that an adverse reaction to a food is automatically an allergic reaction. This is not strictly true. An allergy involves the body's immune system, whereas an intolerance does not.

FOOD ALLERGY

When a person has a true food allergy, the body's immune system treats that food (the allergen) as if it is a dangerous alien, like bacteria or a virus. It releases an abnormal antibody that attacks the protein in the offending food. The resultant effect on the body – such as vomiting, diarrhoea, itchy skin rashes, swelling of the face or throat or difficulty in breathing – is called an allergic reaction. Symptoms can develop within minutes after ingestion or may not appear for several hours. In rare, severe cases, anaphylaxis occurs; the sufferer is unable to breathe properly, there is a dramatic reduction in blood pressure and rapid swelling of the mouth and throat. This can lead to severe shock and can be fatal, so medical help must be sought immediately.

True food allergies affect only about 2 per cent of the population in the long term. However, 5–8 per cent of babies and very young children experience some form of allergic reaction to certain foods, which they may grow out of before school age.

If you or anyone in your immediate family has a food allergy, there is an increased chance that your child will have one too. Since it is quite possible to prevent a food allergy occurring in these instances, it is particularly important that you take extra care when you are weaning the child. (See Weaning Your Potentially Allergenic Baby, page 33.)

FOOD INTOLERANCE

A food intolerance or sensitivity is much more common. It can be serious enough to cause a baby or young child not to thrive and grow properly. Also, it can cause many symptoms: severe colic, tummy upsets and flatulence, persistent runny nose coupled with a persistent cough, eczema, itching with or without skin rashes, asthma or wheezing, bloated or swollen stomach, listlessness, hyperactivity, headaches, aching limbs, frequent crying or mood swings, reflux, constipation and many others. However, I must stress that all children get minor ailments such as runny noses and other cold symptoms and, on their own, these are unlikely to be evidence of food allergies or intolerances.

A food intolerance can sometimes be caused by the lack of an essential enzyme in the digestive system, such as lactase, which is needed to digest lactose, the sugar found in milk.

THE MAJOR ALLERGENS

This section contains information on the major allergens, where to find them and how to avoid them.

COWS' MILK

Cows' milk is the most common cause of allergy and intolerance in babies and very young children. The sugar (lactose) contained in milk causes intolerance and the proteins (casein, lactalbumin and lactoglobulin) cause cows' milk allergy.

Lactose intolerance: This is caused when the enzyme, lactase, is not produced in enough quantity in the small intestine; in rare cases it is not produced at all. The body needs lactase to break down lactose into simple sugars so that it can be absorbed. Without it, the lactose passes straight through to the large intestine. Bacteria feed on the unprocessed milk sugar, creating toxins and gas, which cause painful colic, bloating and diarrhoea. The condition is usually inherited.

A child with lactose intolerance can usually cope with some dairy products, especially hard cheeses and yoghurts. Some will also be able to tolerate goats' or sheep's milk; others will react to these in exactly the same way as cows' milk. Trial and error is the only way to work out what suits your child, and there are alternatives to dairy products available, such as soya, pea, oat and rice milks.

Cows' milk allergy: This is usually fairly easy for a doctor to diagnose. If your baby is fed ordinary infant formula and starts to cry a great deal, becomes listless, suffers from colic and, most importantly, fails to gain weight and thrive, it is extremely likely to be caused by an allergy to cows' milk protein. It can also happen when breastfeeding if the mother's diet is very high in cows' milk. Check with your doctor, who is likely to advise a change to a hypoallergenic formula or to the mother's diet.

This is better than using soya or goats' milk formulas because little babies are often allergic to these as well. Goats' milk formulas are usually suitable for older children if they continue to have a milk protein allergy – this is most likely to happen if a child suffers from other allergies too. Remember that adult soya, oat and rice milks are not suitable as they are not nutritionally complete.

Do not cut out cows' milk or other dairy products unless you have been advised to do so by your doctor. Milk and dairy products are highly valuable foods for most children so they should not be removed from the diet unless absolutely necessary. They provide not only protein, fat and carbohydrate to provide energy for growth, but also and essential minerals, particularly calcium for healthy teeth and bones and zinc to help growth and to fight infections, and vitamins A, B and C.

Foods to avoid if allergy or intolerance diagnosed
Obviously, you need to avoid cows' milk itself and all foods made from it, including:
- Butter, margarine and other dairy spreads
- Cheese
- Yoghurt, crème fraîche and fromage frais
- Canned evaporated and condensed milk

- Dried milk
- Buttermilk
- Cream – all types
- Custard
- Ice cream

Children who are lactose intolerant may be able to take some dairy produce so you need to seek professional help and discover what they can eat through trial and error.

Surprise sources: Many commercially produced foods contain hidden ingredients that you do not expect. You will need to read the labels on the following products as they may contain milk:

- Biscuits (cookies)
- Breads of all types
- Breakfast cereals
- Canned and packet soups
- Chocolate
- Crackers
- Crumb- or batter-coated fish, meat, etc.
- Custards
- Doughnuts
- Flavoured crisps (chips)
- Hot dogs
- Instant hot drinks
- Instant mashed potato
- Pancakes
- Pickles, sauces and relishes
- Pie fillings
- Pizzas
- Processed meats, including ham
- Salad cream, salad dressings
- Sausages
- Scones (biscuits)
- Stock cubes
- Sweets (candies)
- Waffles

Hidden milks: Read the labels for any of the following and avoid them if they contain milk products. Those marked with * may or may not contain milk. Note that casein, which is a milk protein, may be tolerated by some children who are lactose intolerant.

- Butter fat/flavour/oil/solids
- Caramel colour*
- Caramel flavouring*
- Casein, hydrolised casein, rennet casein
- Caseinates (ammonium, calcium, magnesium, potassium, sodium)
- Curds
- Dried milk (non-fat milk powder)
- Dry milk solids
- Flavouring*
- High protein flour*
- Hydrolised milk protein
- Lactalbumin, lactalbumin phosphate
- Lactate
- Lactoferrin
- Lactoglobulin
- Lactose
- Milk derivative/fat/solids
- Natural flavouring*
- Non-fat milk/milk solids
- Nougat
- Opta (fat replacer)
- Simplesse (fat replacer)
- Solids
- Soured (dairy sour) cream solids and soured milk solids
- Syrup sweetener
- Whey, delactosed whey, demineralised whey, sweet whey powder, whey powder, whey protein concentrate, whey solids

Safe alternatives to dairy products

Milk: Once your child is two years old or is eating well, you have more choices. Soya milk is the obvious one – if your child can tolerate soya. Alternatively, there are rice milks, oat milks, sunflower milks and nut milks. When possible, choose those that are fortified with calcium. Some children can tolerate goats' and/or sheep's milk too.

Lactose-reduced milk is now readily available in supermarkets. It contains all the other nutrients of regular milk, so is not suitable if your child has a milk protein allergy, but for those with lactose intolerance it may be the best solution.

Cheese: Some children with milk allergies may tolerate goats' and sheep's cheeses, and water buffalo Mozzarella. Children with lactose intolerance may be able to tolerate hard cheeses, such as Cheddar, red Leicester and Parmesan, too. There are soya cheese alternatives (in different styles and flavours) for those who can tolerate them and there are even a few rice-based cheeses although most do contain casein so beware. Alternatively, use my home-made substitutes on pages 178 and 180.

Butter and margarine: Dairy-free vegetable margarine is ideal for anyone on an allergen-free diet. If your child can tolerate soya, pure soya spread is a cheaper alternative. You can also use any vegetable or olive oils. Only use corn and nut oils if your child can tolerate them. White vegetable fat is useful, particularly for making pastry (paste).

Yoghurt: Use soya-based yoghurts, if your child can tolerate them. Alternatively, try sheep's or goats' yoghurt. Children with lactose intolerance can sometimes cope with dairy yoghurt anyway.

Cream: Use a soya cream – there are plenty of alternatives but I found Soya Dream the best – if your child can have soya. Alternatively, there are recipes for nut creams and cream substitute later in the book (see pages 181–3) or you can use commercial coconut cream, unless your child is allergic to nuts.

Tofu
Fermented bean curd, or tofu, is a very versatile protein food for children who can eat soya. Silken tofu is creamy and good for dips, cheesecake recipes, sauces and toppings. Firm tofu can be marinated and used in place of cheese or meat. I haven't used it in this book because so many children cannot tolerate soya but do try it if it is suitable – and your child likes it!

GLUTEN
Gluten is one of the proteins in wheat, barley, rye and, to a lesser extent, oats. The small intestine is responsible for absorbing many nutrients from our food through the villi (fronds) on the intestinal walls. If a child has **coeliac disease**, gluten damages the villi, literally flattening the

fronds so that they cannot absorb the nutrients. Consequently, before diagnosis, coeliacs tend to loose weight and become malnourished due to malabsorption of essential nutrients, debilitated and wasted. Diarrhoea, bone disease and anaemia can also be problems. Once gluten is removed completely from the diet, the villi will eventually become restored and function properly again. Nobody knows how or why this happens, but for many sufferers gluten has to be avoided for life. In babies the illness produces foul-smelling, pale stools, wind, bloating and poor weight gain and growth. This usually happens soon after cereals are introduced at around six months. It needs to be diagnosed by a doctor. It is not advisable to give gluten to babies younger than this as their digestive systems are too immature to cope with it.

There are many conflicting ideas about what can or can't be tolerated. If you have any doubts at all about any foods, check with your gastro-enterologist or contact Coeliac UK (their address is given on page 186). They will send you an updated list regularly.

Foods to avoid if allergy or intolerance diagnosed
Foods marked with * may or may not be suitable – check they state they are gluten-free.
Note: Even if a product states it is gluten-free, it could still contain deglutenised wheat (wheat starch) so you must avoid it if your child is intolerant to all parts of wheat grain. In the same way, if it states it's wheat-free, it may still contain gluten. I once made the mistake of buying an organic wheat-free flour mix, only to discover it contained barley.
- All wheat products (see pages 17–18) plus:
- Barley
- Barley malt
- Brown table sauce
- Caramel colour*
- Malt
- Pure malt extract
- Malt syrup
- Oats
- Oatmeal
- Oat bran

- Oyster sauce
- Pearl barley
- Rice malt
- Rye
- Soy sauce*
- Teriyaki sauce
- Tomato ketchup (catsup)*
- Worcestershire sauce*

Safe alternative grains and flours
- Amaranth
- Arrowroot
- Buckwheat
- Corn and maize in all its forms – unless it, too, causes a reaction
- Gram flour
- Millet
- Potato flour
- Quinoa
- Rice in all its forms – and there are masses to choose from
- Sago
- Soya – unless it also causes a reaction
- Shoyu and tamari sauce
- Tapioca
- Urid flour
- Wild rice
- Yam flour

Note that wheat-free, gluten-free flour mix is now available from all good supermarkets and health food shops or you can make your own (see page 164). For diagnosed coeliacs, it is available on prescription.

Safe alternative commercial foods
Pasta: There are loads of corn, rice and buckwheat pastas available in supermarkets and health food shops. You can also make your own (see recipes on pages 72 and 98). I find the rice ones are most popular with children as the texture is most like ordinary wheat pasta. Corn pastas, in particular, are a bit granular when cooked. Traditional Italian pasta is not suitable for anyone with a gluten allergy or intolerance.

Bread, biscuits (cookies) and cakes: You can buy commercially made gluten-free varieties of all these in supermarkets and health food shops (at a price!) and a few items, like rice cakes, are available everywhere. A cheaper alternative is to make your own – see pages 116–47. Some are available on prescription for diagnosed coeliacs.

Facts you should know
Buckwheat: This is not related to wheat in any way and is safe for everyone to eat.

Chips (fries): Home-cooked chips are fine but bought ones may have an added coating that includes wheat, so read the labels. Those from your local fish and chip shop may be fried in oil previously used to cook the fish in batter and may cause cross-contamination, so they are best avoided.

Hydrolysed vegetable protein: In America, it is recommended that coeliacs avoid this, but there is no evidence, as yet, that it causes problems.

Isomalt: This comes from sugar beet, not barley, and is safe for coeliacs. It has a slightly laxative effect on some people but is unlikely to be consumed in large enough quantities to cause a problem.

Malt flavouring: The small amount used as a flavour enhancer in cornflakes, for instance, is safe for most coeliacs. I have therefore called for ordinary cornflakes and rice crispies but if you think your child may be extra-sensitive (check with your gastro-enterologist), you can buy gluten-free varieties in health food shops. Coeliacs should avoid malted drinks and pure malt.

Medicines: Most are fine, but if your doctor is prescribing medication for your child, it's worth reminding him of any allergies the child may have. Some vitamin supplements may contain wheat flour or starch as a filler – if in doubt, check with your pharmacist. On the whole, if a medicine upsets your child's stomach, it is more likely that the medicine itself is causing the problem, rather than any wheat it contains.

Monosodium glutamate: This is a flavour enhancer found in many commercially prepared foods. Although it is made from processed sugar beet and wheat, it is unlikely to cause a reaction in coeliacs or wheat intolerance sufferers. It is, however, high in salt, which is not good for any child (or older person). Try to avoid monosodium glutamate whenever possible. It is often accused by some of causing hyperactivity.

Oats: There is some controversy as to whether oats and oat products do affect coeliacs. Because of the uncertainty, I have excluded them from the main recipes, but they are offered as an alternative for those who can eat them.

Play dough: Commercial and ordinary home-made varieties are made largely from wheat flour. Bought play dough smells nice, so do make sure coeliac children do not nibble at it! (Home-made dough usually has a huge amount of salt in it, which puts children off.) Make sure they wash their hands well after use. As a safe alternative, make my gluten-free, wheat-free version (see page 185).

Quorn: This is a vegetable protein made from a fungus. Plain Quorn in any form is safe. However, ready-prepared meals made with Quorn, either coated or in a sauce, may contain gluten so are not suitable. Note, too, that Quorn is bound with egg albumen, so if your child is allergic to eggs, it should be avoided.

Soya protein: TVP (textured vegetable protein) is safe, as is tofu (soya bean curd). But, if your child is allergic to soya products, then you should avoid these.

Stamps, gummed labels, sticky coloured shapes and envelopes: It is a myth that the gum used contains gluten – your child can safely lick them.

Toothpastes and mouthwashes: The British Dental Association says they are safe. The cellulose gum used as a thickener is gluten-free. However, put only a pea-sized blob of toothpaste on your child's brush and encourage him to rinse his mouth well after use.

Vinegar: Wine, fruit and cider vinegars are fine. There is some controversy about malt and spirit vinegars and for this reason, I have avoided using them in the book. If in any doubt, check with your gastro-enterologist. If your child cannot tolerate them, you will need to check labels of all pickles, dressing and relishes. See pages 166–71 for some delicious recipes for these items.

Yeast: Some baking yeast is cultivated on a wheat substrate (the substance on which the enzyme grows). You may need to phone the manufacturer of your normal brand to check. Alternatively, you can purchase wheat-free yeast from a health food shop.

Always read the labels and make a note of which brands you can use. For instance, Heinz baked beans and tomato ketchup (catsup) are fine for coeliacs, but some other brands are not. Once you've found some established brands, remember that recipes change from time to time – so do continue to read the labels.

WHEAT
In wheat intolerance, the grain itself causes problems. In some ways it's easier than gluten intolerance because your child can, at least, enjoy barley, rye and oats as well as other grains, and unlike sufferers of coeliac disease, there is a good chance your child may grow out of the problem. Even older people who become wheat intolerant in later life can sometimes rebuild their tolerance levels after excluding the culprit for quite a while.

Foods to avoid if allergy or intolerance diagnosed
You will need to read the labels of everything from baked beans to packet desserts. Foods marked with * show that some brands **may** contain wheat in one form or another.
- Abyssinian hard wheat
- Baking powder, unless labelled gluten-free – some have wheat flour added as an anti-clumping agent
- Blue cheese made with breadcrumbs, e.g. Roquefort – the types made with penicillin are fine
- Bread made with wheat flour, including naan, chappatis, pittas, tortillas, rye bread
- Breakfast cereals made with wheat, including muesli
- Brown flour
- Bulgar (cracked wheat)
- Cereal binders
- Chinese egg noodles
- Citric acid – some brands are made from wheat

- Couscous
- Dextrins*
- Durum wheat
- Edible starch*
- Einkorn wheat
- Filler
- Fu (dried wheat gluten)
- Ground spices – they may contain wheat flour
- Gum base
- Hard wheat
- Kamut (pasta wheat)
- Liquorice sweets – liquorice flavouring is fine
- Miso*
- Modified food starch*
- Mono and diglycerides*
- Mustard powder
- Pasta made with wheat
- Semolina (cream of wheat)
- Sodium caseinate
- Soy sauce*
- Spelt (manna)
- Stock cubes*
- Suet in packets – some are coated in wheat flour, others in rice flour (use grated hard white vegetable fat instead)
- Triticale
- Udon (wheat noodles)
- Wheat bran
- Wheat flours – plain (all-purpose), self-raising (self-rising), strong (bread), wholemeal, granary
- Wheatgerm
- Wheat nuts

Safe alternatives to wheat
You can eat all the alternative grains suitable for coeliacs (see page 14) plus:
- Barley – including things like malt flavourings, made from barley
- Oats
- Rye – including pumpernickel and whole rye crispbreads

Note: Many oat, barley or rye breads, biscuits (cookies) and cakes also contain wheat flour, so do read the labels.

EGGS

Egg allergy is most common in babies. It is far more rare in older children as around 80–90 per cent of babies grow out of egg allergy. Reaction is usually an immediate, alarming swelling around the mouth. You need to consult your doctor for advice as it can develop into a more severe allergy and needs proper diagnosis. Eggs are a good source, not only of protein, but also of fat, essential vitamins and minerals. Although it is unwise to give raw or soft-cooked eggs to babies or young children, only avoid cooked eggs if there is a genuine problem. Your doctor may advise you to avoid eggs altogether; to avoid egg whites until the baby is a year old, as the protein in egg white is usually the problem; or, rarely, to avoid egg yolks, in which case you can substitute two egg whites for every whole egg.

Note: Until recently, children with egg allergy could not have the MMR jab because it was grown in egg albumen. This has now changed and in most cases it is perfectly safe for children with such an allergy to have the vaccination. The influenza vaccine may be grown in egg albumen.

Foods to avoid if allergy or intolerance diagnosed
This is not a comprehensive list because eggs are used in so many made-up dishes.

- Batters
- Biscuits (cookies)
- Breads
- Burgers
- Cakes
- Cream fillings
- Crumb-coated meat, fish, poultry
- Custards
- Egg-based sauces e.g. Hollandaise, Tartare
- French toast
- Golden-glazed pastries
- Ice cream
- Macaroons
- Mayonnaise
- Meatballs
- Meringues
- Mousses
- Pancakes

- Pasta made with eggs
- Puddings
- Quorn – it is bound with egg albumen
- Rissoles
- Salad cream
- Soufflés
- Sweet pastries

Some ingredients may not be immediately obvious as indicating eggs. Again you must read the labels and look out the hidden enemy.
- Albumen
- Conalbumin
- Dried egg
- Egg derivatives/substitutes
- Globulin
- Lecithin (E322) – this may be from an egg source so should be avoided unless the source is stated
- Livetin
- Mucoid
- Ovalbumin
- Ovomucoid
- Pasteurised egg
- Vitellin

Using egg replacer
There are two different types of commercial egg replacer on the market. The first type is made from potato starch and tapioca flour with vegetable gum and raising agents. It is mixed with water and can be used for baking, batters, pie fillings and custards. In my recipes, I have used No Egg, because it is totally allergen-free; it may be available to you on prescription. 5 ml/1 tsp to 30 ml/2 tbsp of water is equivalent to 1 egg. You whisk them together until foamy, then use the mixture more or less like normal eggs. Follow the directions in each recipe. There is also an omelette powder in the same range.

The second type is made from soy protein, potato starch and stabiliser and is really only suitable for baking. You need 20 g/³/₄ oz of egg replacer and 80 ml/a generous 5 tbsp of water for every egg. Mix the replacer with the dry ingredients (or creamed fat and sugar) in a recipe, then add the water at the end.

Egg substitutes

If you need to omit whole eggs, you can either use egg replacer (see above) or one of the alternatives below.

As a raising agent: Substitute 5 ml/1 tsp of baking powder (gluten-free if necessary) for each egg in the recipe and stir in with the dry ingredients before adding any liquid. Increase the liquid content by 30 ml/2 tbsp per egg.

As a binder: Dissolve 5 ml/1 tsp powdered gelatine in 45 ml/ 3 tbsp of hot water per egg. Cool, then freeze briefly until the consistency of egg white. Whisk with a fork until frothy, then use as before. Alternatively, when extra moisture isn't needed, use 10 ml/2 tsp of potato flour for each egg.

To stick on a coating: Use 45 ml/3 tbsp of milk (dairy-free if necessary) per beaten egg instead.

To moisten a mixture, e.g. in a rich cake: Use 50 g/ 2 oz/¼ cup of puréed apple (apple sauce).

To be used hard-boiled (hard-cooked) and chopped: Use 50 g/2 oz/¼ cup of crumbled firm tofu (unless your child is allergic to soya protein). Alternatively, use the same quantity of cooked cannellini beans, drained and roughly chopped or mashed.

SOYA BEANS

These are used to make numerous dairy and meat substitutes as well as flavourings, such as soy sauce. Unfortunately, babies who are allergic to cows' milk protein may be allergic to soya formula too. This usually manifests itself when they are transferred from ordinary infant formula on to a soya formula. The symptoms are similar. If it occurs, you will have to change to one of the hypoallergenic formulas. Older children with different food allergies are often allergic to soya milk and other soya products too, which will then have to be avoided. But don't just assume that if your child is allergic to dairy products he will definitely be allergic to soya foods. It isn't always the case and soya products are the simplest and most varied substitutes for dairy products. So discuss the problem with your specialist and try them with caution.

Foods to avoid if allergy or intolerance diagonsed
Ingredients marked with * may or may not contain soya.
- Hot dogs
- Miso (soya bean paste)
- Soy sauce
- Soya beans
- Soya products, e.g. milk, yoghurt, cheeses, margarine
- Tofu
- Veggie burgers
- Worcestershire sauce*

Hidden ingredients
Ingredients marked with * may or may not contain soya.
- De-fatted soya flour
- Hydrolysed vegetable protein*
- Soya bean oil (and foods cooked in it)
- Soya lecithin (E322)
- Soya flour
- Soya grits
- Soya protein
- Soya protein concentrate
- Soya protein isolate
- Textured soya
- Textured vegetable protein*

FISH AND SHELLFISH
An allergy to fish and shellfish tends to affect older children and adults rather than babies. It is rare, but can cause anaphylaxis (see page 7). If, therefore, you think your child is at heightened risk (because of a known allergy in the immediate family), don't give fish to him until he is at least a year old. Shellfish should be avoided until he is at least two. However, you should only avoid fish if it is absolutely necessary as it is a valuable source of protein, essential fatty acids, vitamins and minerals for most children. It is also easily digested (especially when poached or steamed) and its soft texture is enjoyed by most babies – baby fish pie made with mashed white fish, potato and carrots, moistened with a little expressed breast milk or formula is a baby's gourmet delight!

If there is a problem, fish is easy to avoid, as it is not a hidden ingredient in manufactured foods.

PEANUTS

Peanuts (groundnuts) are not really nuts because they don't grow on trees. They are legumes (part of the pea and bean family). Peanut allergy is still rare but is intense. If anyone in your immediate family has a food allergy – and especially a peanut allergy – avoid giving peanuts to your child, even in oil form (although research suggests that refined peanut oil may be acceptable), until he is at least three years old. If your child is allergic to peanuts, even a minute amount can cause anaphylaxis (see page 7). Therefore you have to be vigilant to make sure that every food is peanut-free.

Avoid any foods that may contain nuts of any kind – there is no way of telling if they are peanuts and you can't afford to take a chance. This means never buying unwrapped bread or cakes from a bakery or food from a delicatessen (as cross-contamination is very likely). Only buy products that are pre-packed and declared 'nut-free'. I must stress, though, that peanuts are a valuable source of protein for most children. Smooth peanut butter is particularly useful.

Note: Children who are allergic to peanuts may be able to eat other varieties of nuts that grow on trees (e.g. walnuts, almonds, etc.) The two allergies are not the same. However, if a child is allergic to peanuts, the usual advice is that all nuts should be avoided. Children under five years of age should not be given whole peanuts as they could cause choking. Unfortunately, nut allergies don't usually go away.

Foods to avoid if allergy or intolerance diagnosed
- All unpackaged baked goods that may contain a trace of peanuts
- Any foods labelled with a warning that they might contain a trace of nuts
- Ethnic foods, e.g. Thai, Asian and Indonesian
- Groundnut oil
- Mixed nuts
- Peanuts and peanut butter
- Sweets that may contain peanuts

TREE NUTS

An allergy to tree nuts is even more rare than peanut allergy and is not necessarily linked to it. A reaction will be caused by any nuts in hard shells such as walnuts, brazil nuts, hazelnuts (filberts), pecans and almonds. Coconut is unlikely to cause a reaction. It may also include seeds, such as sesame seeds. As with peanuts, the reaction time may be swift and intense and can cause anaphylaxis. Again, like peanuts, tree nuts are a valuable source of protein for most children, so don't avoid them unless you have to. Do not give nuts or seeds to the very young, with or without allergies, as they could choke.

Foods to avoid if allergy or intolerance diagnosed
- All foods that declare there may be a trace of nuts in them
- All foods visibly containing nuts
- All unrefined nut oils, e.g. sesame, walnut
- All sweets (candies) that could contain nuts
- Baked goods that could have hidden nuts, e.g. ground almonds or almond essence (extract) in a cake.
- Baked goods that may have been in contact with nuts

MINOR ALLERGENS

As well as the common allergens listed above, there are other foods that can cause symptoms of intolerance or allergy in a much smaller number of people. These include corn, tomatoes, strawberries and citrus fruits. All are valuable and tasty foods for most children so, as the number of children having to avoid them is so small, I've included them in the recipes, together with a substitute in the recipe introduction. Very occasionally, any other food, such as apples, cherries or celery, may cause a reaction but it is so unusual that I offer the advice just as a warning, not implying that they are serious allergen contenders. Sugar does not cause allergies but should be kept to a minimum to prevent obesity and dental problems.

Yeast allergy is so very rare I have not included it in this book. It is extremely difficult to deal with and if you suspect your child has a yeast allergy you will need proper supervision from a hospital dietician. The list of things that must be excluded from the diet is very long. It includes anything made with yeast, including all breads, pizzas and cakes; yeast extract (Marmite or Vegemite); anything that is fermented, like soy sauce, tofu, vinegar; and anything that includes the skin of fresh fruit, such as sugary spreads and jams (conserves). You will also be told to reduce the amount of sugar in the diet, to prevent the natural growth of yeast cells within the digestive system.

IDENTIFYING THE CULPRIT

Before you can take any kind of action, you need to establish what it is that is causing your child's allergic or intolerant symptoms. As I've said before, recognising cows' milk allergy may become obvious when you try giving your child infant formula or when transferring from breast to follow-on milk or cows' milk. Gluten intolerance can also be fairly easily identified (see page 13). Severe symptoms, like anaphylaxis, won't pass you by but food intolerances, for the most part, are more difficult to pin-point. If you suspect a food allergy or intolerance, there are some things you can do to make it easier to spot.

A baby must be supervised by a health professional. You will probably be advised to introduce new foods only one at a time, four to five days apart. That way, if there is an adverse reaction, you will know exactly which food is causing it. Any adverse reaction should be noted and the food avoided until you have checked with your doctor or health visitor. Keep a diary for future reference.

With an older child, who is eating complete, regular meals, it is more difficult. Try keeping a diary for a week or two and seek a dietician's advice. Write down everything he eats, making a special note of any new foods, and noting when symptoms develop. With any luck, when you analyse the results, you will find that you can pick out which food or ingredient is causing the problem. Then try eliminating the suspected food or ingredient for a week or two and observe the results.

Note: Do not cut out different foods willy-nilly. You must make sure your child is getting the right balance of nutrients (see Happy, Healthy Eating, pages 28–31). You must substitute a suitable alternative for key foods such as dairy products and wheat.

Remember that your child may not have been born with an intolerance. It can take weeks, months or even years to build up enough to cause noticeable symptoms. However, just because your child is off-colour does not necessarily mean he is developing an intolerance.

MEDICAL HELP AND ADVICE

If you do suspect your baby or child has a serious allergy or intolerance, you must seek immediate medical advice. See your GP, paediatrician or health visitor. Some members of the medical profession are sympathetic, others not quite so responsive. To test for an allergy, they may give him a skin prick test or a blood test and recommend an exclusion diet and reintroduction of foods recorded in a diary. For an intolerance, no other test has a scientific basis other than the exclusion and reintroduction diet and diary. Do not be tempted to visit your health food shop or chemist for an allergy test. These have no scientific basis and are likely to maldiagnose.

Your doctor will be able to give your child medication to help him cope with breathing problems and he will also prescribe antihistamines for itching, rashes, etc. Don't be alarmed if he suggests steroid creams – those prescribed for babies and young children are specially formulated to be very mild and the relief they give your child will be almost immediate.

If your child is anaphylactic, you will be advised to purchase a special bracelet for him to wear, which is engraved with details of the problem. You will also be provided with a special pen called an EpiPen (epinephrine autoinjection device) or Anapen so he can be given a very quick injection of adrenaline to prevent anaphylactic shock if he inadvertently comes into contact with an allergen.

PROTECTING YOUR CHILD AS HE GROWS

Many children outgrow their allergies before they need to take responsibility for their own well-being. But for children who continue to have problems as they grow older, it is very important that they are educated to know what they can and can't eat when they are away from home. There are also a few other precautions you can take to ensure your child's safety when you are not around.

- Make their friends, friends' parents and teachers aware of their problem and how to deal with it and provide regular updates.
- If your child is anaphylactic, make sure he wears his medical alert bracelet at all times and never forgets to

carry his EpiPen. You may find his nursery or school will also be prepared to keep one handy.

• Teach your child to read labels on foods, to check the ingredients for potential allergens.

Going to parties can bring problems. If necessary, give your child a 'goody bag' with his own party food in it – and try to make it fun party food (see the recipes on pages 148–62 and buy special treats). If necessary, make a quantity of the party treats and donate them so other children can enjoy them too (just make sure you remind the organiser to make sure your child eats only the suitable goodies).

FOOD ADDITIVES

There is huge controversy over the use of food additives. Some additives are necessary for preserving foods, others add flavour with no ill-effects whatsoever. Most are considered safe and are regulated by law but different countries have different regulations and whereas some additives have been banned universally, others are allowed in some countries. The UK is governed by EU rules and all food additives have been rigorously tested before they are allowed in our foods. But many parents still find that their children do react to certain colourings, flavourings or preservatives and so if you notice that your child does react to a particular E-number, then make sure that you avoid buying foods or drinks containing it.

More research is needed to find concrete evidence of links between additives and allergies but some scientists have discovered an association between certain colourings – particularly tartrazine (E102) – and asthma, migraine and hyperactivity in children. In addition, some preservatives, particularly benzoates and sulphites (E210–227), can cause problems for severe asthmatics. If your child has an adverse reaction to a product containing any of these E-numbers, you will have to buy organic brands. Since one of the items involved is wine vinegar, this may mean cutting out lots of pickles and condiments.

Of course, it's probably not a good idea for any of us to consume chemicals that we don't need, so it makes sense to avoid foods that contain them when possible.

HAPPY, HEALTHY EATING

Whether you are making your own baby food, or buying ready-made cans or jars, you need to be sure that the meals you provide contain everything your child needs in order to grow. If you are preparing your own food, particularly for small babies, you must also take great care with hygiene.

A BALANCED DIET

Every child needs a balanced diet. Breast milk or formula (if necessary) provides vital nutrients for growing babies until they are at least a year old. But when your child has been weaned on to solid food, it is up to you to ensure he gets all the nutrients he needs from the different food groups. Remember, his needs are not exactly the same as yours. He may be small but because he is growing so fast he needs a huge amount of energy in comparison to you in the form of a much higher fat and protein intake as well as a good carbohydrate supply.

FATS

Unlike adults, your child should get almost 50 per cent of his calories from fat in the first year, then about 35 per cent up to 5 years of age. This will be largely from milk, at first, but he will also need to eat a mixture of fats. If he is allergic to dairy products and eggs, this causes great problems as they are the main sources of the foods he needs. To make sure he gets the fat he requires, use dairy-free margarine in cooking and as a spread; give him lean meat (there is fat in the tissues), fish (unless he is allergic to it), calcium-enriched dairy-free milks (soya, nut, rice, etc., according to his needs), vegetable oils and white vegetable fat and hydrogenated oils and fats, found in biscuits (cookies) and cakes – even commercially prepared gluten-free ones. There is also some fat in cereals. The essential fatty acids found in oily fish, plant oils and nuts are vital for the development of the brain. If your child has to omit one of these sources, try to compensate with more of the other foods.

PROTEINS

These are vital for your baby's growth and development. Breast milk or formula (where necessary) will provide the main source at first. Then, when your baby is weaned, the proteins will come from meat, poultry, fish, some vegetables, such as dried peas, beans and lentils, and dairy products. If your child is allergic to any of these, you must provide alternatives. Cereals, nuts, seeds and soya products can be valuable sources (although not all children can tolerate them) and useful fruit sources include avocados and bananas. It should be noted that vegetable proteins, unless of soya origin, do not have the same high protein content, so don't avoid meat, poultry, fish and dairy products unless absolutely necessary.

CARBOHYDRATES

These provide a lot of your child's energy (calories). There are two types. Complex carbohydrates are the starches that fill us up, like potatoes, sweet potatoes, yams, bananas, bread (made from wheat or other grains), cereals, pasta (from wheat, rice, millet or other grains), rice, polenta, couscous and bulgar (cracked wheat). Simple carbohydrates are the refined sugars that are found in so many processed foods. They are known as 'empty calories', because they contain only energy and no other nutrients and they can cause dental cavities, obesity and other complications. However, they do add palatability. Young babies do not need added sugar at all. It just encourages them to develop a sweet tooth (something they are not born with). Avoid sour foods in the early days, so you are not tempted to sweeten them. Of course, as children grow up, they will start to eat some foods, such as cooking (tart) apples, that could not be enjoyed without sweetener. In this case, I would suggest sweetening with dried fruits (note, though, that these can also cause tooth cavities if given in excess), or a little honey – as it is sweeter than sugar, you don't need much and, unlike sugar, it does contain some trace vitamins and minerals. In my recipes, I have used some refined sugar, particularly in baking and for special treat foods, but only when it is necessary for palatable results.

VITAMINS AND MINERALS

These are found in all fresh foods. Fruit and vegetables are the main suppliers.

Vitamin A (including retinal and beta-carotene): Vital for healthy bones, vision and skin and for growth and fighting infection. It is found in liver, eggs, and naturally red, orange and yellow fruit and vegetables, such as sweet potatoes, sweetcorn (corn), mangoes, yellow and red (bell) peppers, peaches and tomatoes.

B group vitamins (including folate): Vital for the development of the nervous system and for growth and good digestion. These are found in lean meat, soya products, oily fish, green leafy vegetables, dairy produce, wholegrain cereals (all types), Marmite or other yeast extract, bananas, avocados and nuts.

Vitamin C: Vital for growth and repair of all body tissues. It also helps your child absorb iron. It is found in green leafy vegetables, black and red currants, kiwi fruit, potatoes (just under the skin so peel thinly or scrub and cook with the skin on), (bell) peppers, citrus fruit and strawberries. There is also some in most other fruits.

Vitamin D: Important for healthy bones and teeth. It is used to absorb calcium and phosphorus and is made by the body when it is exposed to sunlight. It is also found in oily fish, such as tuna and salmon, and dairy products and eggs. Although these are all potential allergens, it is vital that you don't deprive your child of any of them unless essential.

Vitamin E: Vital for well-being and cell growth. The best sources are vegetable oils, avocados, nuts and wheat germ.

Calcium: Essential for healthy teeth and bones. This is most readily available in cows' milk and dairy produce, but also in leafy vegetables, tofu and other soya products, oily fish (especially in the soft bones of canned salmon or sardines, so mash them thoroughly with the food for toddlers and older children), nuts and seeds. If your child is allergic to calcium-rich foods, make sure he has a calcium-enriched milk substitute. For children between the ages of one and five, 450 ml/³/₄ pt/2 cups of milk or enriched milk substitute provides the daily requirement of calcium.

Iron: Vital for growth and well-being. A lack of iron leads to anaemia, listlessness and potential illness. Babies are born with enough iron to last for their first six months of life. After that they need to get it from bread (of different grains), fortified baby rice and breakfast cereals, liver, oily fish, red meat, green, leafy vegetables, dried fruits and pulses. Other minerals are needed in very small quantities and, if your child eats a varied diet, he should get enough.

SUPPLEMENTS

Most children on a well-balanced diet do not need supplements. However, you will have noticed that the lists above contain many food items that are potential allergens, so if your child is suffering from severe food allergies, it may be a good idea to give him extra vitamins and minerals in supplement form. Check with your doctor or health visitor. Vitamin drops are available to add to your baby's milk or any other suitable drink.

FIBRE

Although babies and children do not need as much fibre as adults, they do need some to keep their bowel motions regular. But children under two years of age should not be given large quantities of high-fibre foods, such as brown rice, whole grains or bran. Their immature digestive systems cannot cope with them, they prevent the absorption of iron, calcium and other essential nutrients, and also too much fibre fills them up so they do not eat properly, so losing required nutrients.

If your baby gets constipated (which is quite common during weaning), increase his intake of fruits and vegetables and offer more boiled, cooled water.

GOOD HYGIENE

Good general cleanliness is essential when preparing food for babies and young children.

- Sterilise all bottles, teats and feeder cups until your baby is a year old. Sterilise spoons at first, too.
- Always wash and dry your baby's food bowls in hot, soapy water, then rinse and dry on a scrupulously clean tea towel (dish cloth), or use the dishwasher.
- Always wash your hands before preparing food.

- Always wash and dry fresh produce before use.
- Don't lick your fingers and use a clean spoon every time you taste the food.
- Don't put raw and cooked meat on the same shelf in the fridge. Store raw meat on a plate on the bottom shelf, so it can't drip over other foods. Keep all perishable foods wrapped separately. Don't overfill the fridge or it will remain too warm.
- Never use a cloth to wipe down a chopping board you have been using for cutting up meat, for instance, then use the same one to wipe down your work surfaces – you will simply spread germs. Always wash your cloth well in hot, soapy water and, ideally, use an anti-bacterial kitchen cleaner on all surfaces too.
- Do not give out-of-date or reheated foods.

Storing and reheating food
- Transfer leftovers to a clean container and cover with a lid, clingfilm (plastic wrap) or foil. Cool completely, then store in the fridge. Use within two days.
- Never put any warm food in the fridge.
- Do not leave food lying around in the warm kitchen once it is cold.
- If preparing baby food for the freezer, cover and let it cool completely, then freeze as soon as possible.
- Don't re-freeze foods that have defrosted unless you cook them first.
- When reheating food, always make sure it is piping hot throughout, never just lukewarm.
- Never reheat previously cooked food more than once.

FREEZER STORAGE TIMES

Bread and cakes	2 months
Breast milk (expressed either for spare feeds or to moisten baby foods)	1 month
Chicken pieces	1 month
Fish dishes, cooked	3 months
Meat and poultry dishes, cooked	3 months
Sausages and burgers, raw	1 month
Vegetable dishes, cooked	6 months
Vegetable purées	6 months
Fruit purées	6 months

WEANING YOUR POTENTIALLY ALLERGENIC BABY

I must stress here and now that if there is no incidence of food allergy in the immediate family, this chapter does not apply to you. It is intended solely for parents who **know** that their baby is at an increased risk of allergies, for example because of a family history of eczema, asthma, hayfever, rhinitis or food allergy, or other known medical condition. If this is not the case, you should never be tempted to deprive your child of important nutrients – such as cows' milk – just because they are potential allergens for some people. You will be doing your child far more harm than good by stopping him eating these nutritious foods.

FEEDING A HIGH-RISK BABY

If you or anyone else in your immediate family does have a food allergy, your baby is at much higher risk of developing one too, especially if the baby's mother has the allergy. However, there are several steps you can take to try to prevent this happening.

Remember: you should only follow these rules if your child is potentially allergenic. Always seek advice from your GP or health visitor.

- If you are breastfeeding your baby, avoid 'topping up' with infant formula. Breast milk will give your baby the best possible immunity to allergies but formula may interfere with this. In extremely rare cases, your baby may start to show allergic reactions whilst on breast milk alone. If this should happen, it means he may be reacting to something he is absorbing through the breast milk so you should seek medical advice and may need to omit potential allergens from your own diet.
- If you do have to supplement or cannot breastfeed successfully, be aware that normal formula is made

from modified cows' milk and might cause an adverse reaction. Soya or goats' milk formula may have a similar effect. If your baby does react, ask your GP if you should change to a hypoallergenic formula.

- Don't start your baby on solids until he is at least six months old, and continue breastfeeding during weaning. Use iron-fortified baby rice as a first taster. Start by offering just a small spoonful of baby rice, mixed with expressed breast milk (or formula if you are using it) at a feed when your baby seems most hungry.
- There is some evidence that delaying giving potential allergens – such as wheat or eggs – to high-risk babies may help prevent an allergic reaction. However, by doing this you could deprive your baby of valuable nutrients unnecessarily, which is **not** a good idea. My advice is to wean your baby in the normal way. When you start offering different foods, introduce one new one only every four to five days. That way, if he has an adverse reaction, you will be able to identify the culprit and take steps accordingly.
- Try to stay relaxed about allergies and only do as much as you can – it may be difficult to follow all this advice. If you become anxious at mealtimes, worried about how your baby will react, he will pick up on the tension and you will have set the scene for problem eating in the future!

WHAT TO DO IF YOUR BABY SUFFERS AN ADVERSE REACTION TO A FOOD

- If your child has a severe reaction or you are concerned in any way, **seek medical help immediately.**
- If it is a fairly mild reaction, identify the culprit and don't offer that food again for three months, then try again. If there is a further reaction, avoid the food altogether until your child is three years old. By then, he may well have grown out of it, so you can try again.
- If you believe your child does have a food allergy or intolerance, tell your health visitor or go to your GP.

As I have said, you should not put your child on to a restricted diet at any stage of weaning unless it is totally necessary and only under medical guidance. The best way to ensure that your baby gets all the nutrients he needs whilst avoiding any potential allergens is to make your own baby food – and it really couldn't be simpler. In most cases, there is no need to cook specially for your baby. You can simply adapt the food you are preparing for the rest of the family.

PURÉES
The first solid food any baby has must be smooth and easy to swallow.

Vegetable purées: Start with individual roots and tubers – potato, parsnip, carrot, sweet potato, swede (rutabaga), etc. When cooking a vegetable for the family meal, boil it without salt, take out a piece for your baby, then season the remainder. If you are cooking specifically for your baby, peel the chosen vegetable and cut it up fairly small. Boil it in the minimum of water or steam it until tender, to retain the maximum nutrients. Do not add salt. Purée the vegetable in a blender or food processor or through a baby mouli machine. If necessary, moisten the purée with a little of the cooking water, or plain boiled water or expressed milk. Store any extra in ice-cube trays for future use. You can then heat a cube or two in a bowl over a pan of simmering water or in the microwave to serve on its own or heat several different ones as a mixture when your baby has acquired a few more tastes.

Once your baby is used to his root vegetable purée, you can introduce other vegetables, like brassicas, vegetable fruits and so on. Stronger flavours – such as cauliflower – may be made blander to begin with, by mixing the purée with a little baby rice as well as liquid.

Cooked fruit purées: Stew sweet, soft fruits, such as eating (dessert) apples or ripe plums with the tough skin removed, on their own or with a little water. Do not add sugar. If you think a fruit is too sour, mix it with some mashed banana.

Raw fruit purées: Mushy fruits, such as bananas and avocados, can be mashed thoroughly with a fork. Try peeling some skin off an eating (dessert) apple and then scraping off the flesh with a teaspoon – this is very useful if you are out and your baby needs a quick snack.

Mixed protein and vegetable purées: When the vegetables and fruit are established in your baby's diet – at about eight months – you can introduce proteins. Purée a little poached or stewed chicken, red meat, liver or fish fillet (make sure there are absolutely no bones) with a little potato or other vegetable. Remember not to add any dairy products yet. Avoid cured or salted meats or fish until your baby is at least one year old and then give only in very small quantities. Your baby is unlikely to show a reaction to fish now. If it is going to happen, it is more likely to be when he gets a bit older.

ADDING TEXTURE

Once your baby gets used to purées and is cutting teeth, you can progress to a little more texture. Try mashing cooked rice, rice noodles or potato with a little minced (ground) meat or poultry or flaked fish, moistened with a little of the cooking water or expressed milk or formula. Do not add salt to anything. Add a vegetable he likes, too, such as mashed carrot. Once he gets used to mashed or minced food, you can finely chop it, gradually leaving larger chunks. When you start dairy products (at about one year), you can try mixing grated hard cheese with the vegetable. If you already know your baby is allergic to dairy products, because he couldn't take ordinary formula, try goats' or sheep's cheese, watching for any reaction, or try non-dairy commercial alternatives or home-made ones (see pages 178 and 180).

FINGER FOODS

When your child is ready for finger food, try making tiny sandwiches from wheat-free/gluten-free bread, with a thin scraping of dairy-free margarine and, perhaps a scraping of Marmite or other yeast extract. Suitable fillings include cheese substitute (see my recipe for No-allergen Hard Cheese on page 178) or Apple and Date Spread (see page

179) or mashed banana or avocado. You can also help the pain of teething by letting him gnaw on a wheat-free/gluten-free rusk (see page 126), sticks of carrot (put them in the freezer first to help cool the gums) or wedges of apple, cooled in the fridge before cutting.

WHOLE MEALS

Once you have established a repertoire of foods, your baby will be taking less milk and eating more solids, still mashed or finely chopped. At this point, with any luck, you will have identified which foods he is allergic to and can then omit them from his diet, using the recipes in this book.

DRINKS

Offer cooled, boiled water during meals. You can also give warm milk (non-dairy if necessary), perhaps at breakfast and last thing at night, and water or diluted fresh fruit juice (one part juice to six parts water) as a refreshing drink during the day.

Do not give sugary drinks or undiluted pure fruit juice. If your child is allergic to citrus fruits, you will probably find that apple juice is the most popular.

NOTES ON THE RECIPES

- All ingredients are given in imperial, metric and American measures. Follow one set only in a recipe. American terms are given in brackets.
- All spoon measures are level: 1 tsp=5 ml; 1 tbsp=15 ml
- Use medium eggs unless otherwise stated.
- Always wash, peel, core and seed, if necessary, fresh produce before use.
- Salt and sugar should be kept to a minimum. I have suggested lightly seasoning foods where I think it is appropriate. Ideally, don't add any salt or sugar at all.
- I have called for gluten-free products where some brands are not suitable for coeliacs or children on wheat-free diets. If this is not relevant to your child, use ordinary ingredients (e.g. baked beans, Worcestershire sauce or baking powder).
- I have also called for dairy-free/gluten-free **vegetable** stock cubes because they are the most readily available (I use a brand called Kallo, but there are others). However, you can buy gluten-free (but not dairy-free) meat and chicken stock cubes, so use in place of the vegetable ones where appropriate if you prefer.
- Always use fresh herbs unless dried are specifically called for. If you wish to substitute dried for fresh, use only half the quantity or less, as they are very pungent. Frozen, chopped varieties have a better flavour than the dried ones.
- All can sizes are approximate as they vary from brand to brand. For example, if I call for a 400 g/14 oz/large can of tomatoes and yours is a 397 g can, that's fine.
- I have called for dairy-free margarine and milk. Use whichever type suits your child.
- In the substitutes, if your child can tolerate dairy products I have suggested using whole milk for under-5s, semi-skimmed for older children. Obviously, if you are cooking for the whole family, you can use semi-skimmed for everyone, as long as you make sure your pre-schooler gets enough whole milk to drink during the day.

- In the UK, golden syrup is made from cane or beet sugar. In the US, the equivalent (known as light corn syrup) is made from corn. This obviously cannot be given to children with a corn allergy, so I have suggested maple syrup or clear honey as alternatives.
- Cooking times are approximate and should be used as a guide only. Always check that food is thoroughly cooked through before serving.

USING THE SYMBOLS

All the recipes in this book have been carefully formulated to exclude all the major allergens so that they will suit children with multiple allergies as well as those with one specific problem. However, most children aren't allergic to everything, so you will want to use ordinary ingredients where your child can tolerate them. To help you do this, I have offered variations that may be used instead of the allergen-free ingredients to suit your child's requirements and tastes.

Where ingredients may be substituted, they are marked with an appropriate symbol:

   ⊂⊃ = Eggs
   🍶 = Dairy
   ＼ = Wheat
   🌾 = Oats
   ☙ = Soya
   ◉ = Nuts
   🐟 = Fish

So, for example, if your child can tolerate eggs, look for the ⊂⊃ symbol in the ingredients list and then check the Variations box for instructions on how to alter the recipe to include eggs.

BREAKFASTS

It can be difficult to persuade children to eat breakfast and those with food allergies obviously have less variety to choose from. However, it is important that your child gets a nourishing breakfast to set him up for the day ahead. This section offers a whole range of tasty, tempting, nourishing breakfast dishes – from cereals to sausages – that will suit all members of the family.

Many cereals contain wheat or gluten – but see the box on the next page for useful tips. Eggs are not suitable for some and, although there are good alternatives to dairy products, milk or milk products are often hidden in commercial products (again, see next page).

BREAKFAST CEREALS

If your child is coeliac, he should still be able to eat rice crispies or cornflakes. Although they contain malt flavouring, the small amount does not affect most sufferers. There are specific gluten-free varieties in health food shops if your child is one of the few who can't tolerate this.

Instant oat cereal (not suitable for coeliacs) is excellent for most babies over six months, but for potentially allergenic babies, wait until eight months.

Those on a dairy-free regime should read labels carefully. Many flavoured cereals and mueslis contain milk in one form or another. You can buy millet, buckwheat and quinoa grains in health food shops and by mail order (see page 186) and these are very useful in all kinds of recipes.

Fluffy Buckwheat Pancakes

If your child is allergic to corn, you should not give him American light corn syrup – offer maple syrup instead.

MAKES ABOUT 12

150 g/5 oz/ 1¼ cups buckwheat flour ⬟ ☉

25 g/1 oz/¼ cup potato flour ☉

15 ml/1 tbsp gluten-free baking powder

A good pinch of salt

25 g/1 oz/2 tbsp caster (superfine) sugar

375 ml/13 fl oz /1½ cups dairy-free milk ▼

Sunflower oil, for cooking

Golden (light corn) syrup, to serve

1 Mix the flours, baking powder, salt and sugar in a bowl. Beat in the milk to make a smooth batter.

2 Heat a little oil in a frying pan (skillet). Add 30 ml/ 2 tbsp of the batter, spread round to make a small pancake and cook until risen and golden underneath. Flip over and cook the other side until golden. Slide on to a plate and keep warm while cooking the remainder.

3 Serve hot with syrup.

Tolerant to ...	Variations
⬟ Wheat	Use wholemeal flour or half wholemeal, half plain (all-purpose) flour instead of the buckwheat, for a change.
☉ Eggs	Increase the buckwheat (or ordinary flour) to 175 g/6 oz/1½ cups and omit the potato flour. Use 2 eggs, lightly beaten, and reduce the milk to 300 ml/½ pt/1¼ cups. Beat the eggs into the flour mixture with half the milk, then stir in the remaining milk.
▼ Dairy	Use cows' milk – full-cream for under-5s, semi-skimmed for older children.

French Toast Fingers with Fruit Dip

SERVES 1

1 small banana

1 nectarine, peach or pear

A squeeze of lemon juice (optional)

1–2 slices of wheat-free/gluten-free bread
(see pages 117–24) ✎

30–60 ml/2–4 tbsp dairy-free milk 🍶 ⌒

A little sunflower oil, for cooking

10–15 ml/¹/₂–1 tbsp caster (superfine) sugar

A good pinch of ground cinnamon

1 Peel and slice the banana, then put in a blender or food processor. Peel the peach, nectarine or pear, halve, remove the stone (pit) or core, cut into pieces and add to the banana. Add a few drops of lemon juice and run the machine until smooth. Pour into a small bowl on a plate.

2 Dip the bread in the milk.

3 Heat enough oil to cover the base of a frying pan (skillet). Fry (sauté) the bread until golden on both sides. Drain on kitchen paper (paper towels).

4 Meanwhile, mix the sugar and cinnamon on a plate. Dip the fried bread in the sugar mixture to coat on both sides. Cut into fingers.

5 Arrange the fingers around the bowl of fruit purée and serve. Dip the fingers in the purée to eat it. Eat any remainder with a spoon.

Tolerant to ...	Variations
Dairy	Use cows' milk – full-cream for under-5s, semi-skimmed for older children.
Eggs	Use a beaten egg and half the given quantity of milk, either dairy or not, according to allergies.
Wheat	Use ordinary bread.

Quinoa Porridge

SERVES 1

25 g/1 oz/¼ cup quinoa

200 ml/7 fl oz/scant 1 cup water or dairy-free milk

A pinch of salt

Sugar or honey, to taste

Dairy-free milk or cream substitute (see pages 181–3), to serve

1 Wash the quinoa thoroughly in a sieve (strainer). Drain and tip into a non-stick saucepan.

2 Add the water or milk and salt.

3 Bring to the boil, reduce the heat and simmer gently for about 20 minutes until soft and moist.

4 Tip into a serving bowl, sweeten to taste with sugar or honey and serve with a little milk or cream substitute.

Tolerant to ...	Variations
Oats	Use rolled oats instead of quinoa (no need to wash first). Cook for 5 minutes only.
Dairy	Use cows' milk – full-cream for under-5s, semi-skimmed for older children.

Honey Raisin Crunch Cereal

MAKES ABOUT 300 G/12 OZ

175 g/6 oz /1½ cups millet flakes 🌾

50 g/2 oz/⅓ cup raisins ●

60 ml/4 tbsp clear honey

Dairy-free milk, to serve 🥛

1   Put the millet in a heavy-based frying pan (skillet) over a moderate heat.

2   Cook, tossing all the time, for a few minutes until golden brown. Do not allow to burn. Turn the heat to low.

3   Add the raisins and honey and stir until well coated. Cook for about 30 seconds until you can smell the sugar. Take care not to over-brown the mixture or burn the raisins.

4   Tip on to a sheet of non-stick baking parchment and leave to cool.

5   Store in an airtight container. Serve with milk.

Tolerant to ...	Variations
🌾 Oats	Use rolled oats instead of the millet.
● Nuts	Use chopped mixed nuts instead of the raisins and brown with the cereal.
🥛 Dairy	Use cows' milk – full-cream for under-5s, semi-skimmed for older children.

Cherry and Apple Quinoa

SERVES 1

25 g/1 oz/¼ cup quinoa ❀

25 g/1 oz/2 tbsp glacé (candied) cherries

1 eating (dessert) apple, peeled, cored and chopped

200 ml/7 fl oz/scant 1 cup water

Clear honey

Dairy-free milk or cream substitute (see pages 181–3), to serve ❦

1 Rinse the quinoa thoroughly in a sieve (strainer).

2 Tip into a non-stick saucepan and add the cherries, apples and water.

3 Bring to the boil, reduce the heat and simmer gently for about 20 minutes until the grains are soft and moist with most of the liquid is absorbed.

4 Sweeten to taste with honey. Serve in a bowl with a little milk or cream substitute.

Tolerant to ...	Variations
❀ Oats	Use rolled oats instead of quinoa (no need to wash first). Cook for 5 minutes only.
❦ Dairy	Use cows' milk – full-cream for under-5s, semi-skimmed for older children – or ordinary cream.

Apple and Banana Rock Muffins

These have all the goodness of cereal and fruit but in a finger food! You can reheat them briefly in the microwave or oven before serving if liked.

MAKES 12

---

1 large ripe banana

50 g/2 oz/¹⁄₄ cup caster (superfine) sugar

A good pinch of salt

1.5 ml/¹⁄₄ tsp ground cinnamon (optional)

5 ml/1 tsp No Egg egg replacer (see page 20) ⌒

30 ml/2 tbsp warm water

100 g/4 oz/1 cup rice flour ↘

50 g/2 oz/¹⁄₂ cup baby rice cereal ❀

15 ml/1 tbsp gluten-free baking powder

45 ml/3 tbsp sunflower oil

75 ml/5 tbsp cold water

2 eating (dessert) apples, peeled, cored and finely chopped

1 Line 12 sections of a tartlet tin (patty pan) with paper cake cases (cupcake papers).

2 Mash the banana thoroughly or purée in a blender or food processor. Add the sugar, salt, cinnamon and mix again.

3 Whisk the egg replacer with the warm water until frothy. Add to the banana mixture with the rice flour, baby rice, baking powder, oil and cold water. Beat well with a wooden spoon or by running the machine for a few seconds. Stir in the apples.

4 Spoon into the paper cases – they should be full.

5 Bake in a preheated oven at 200°C/400°F/gas mark 6 (fan oven 180°C) for 10–15 minutes until risen, firm and spongy to the touch. Serve warm or cold.

Tolerant to ...	Variations
✎ Wheat	Use plain (all-purpose) or wholemeal flour.
☞ Eggs	Use 1 small egg instead of egg replacer and omit the warm water.
✻ Oats	Use instant oat cereal instead of the baby rice, if liked.

Rice, Buckwheat and Fruit Crisp Cereal

MAKES ABOUT 450 G/1 LB

50 g/2 oz/¼ cup soft light brown sugar

50 g/2 oz/¼ cup dairy-free margarine 🥛

100 g/4 oz/2 cups rice crispies

100 g/4 oz/1 cup buckwheat grains

50 g/2 oz/⅓ cup sultanas (golden raisins)

50 g/2 oz/⅓ cup dried banana chips, roughly crushed

Dairy-free milk, to serve 🥛

1 Melt the sugar and margarine in a large saucepan.

2 Remove from the heat and stir in the cereals and fruits until thoroughly mixed.

3 Spread the mixture out on a baking (cookie) sheet to cool.

4 Store in an airtight container. Serve with milk.

Tolerant to ...	Variations
🥛 Dairy	Use ordinary butter or margarine, and cows' milk – full-cream for under-5s, semi-skimmed for older children.

Plain Breakfast Muffins

Make these in advance, then warm briefly in the microwave or oven before serving.

MAKES 12

---

225 g/8 oz/2 cups wheat-free/gluten-free flour mix ⟍

A pinch of salt

15 ml/1 tbsp gluten-free baking powder

**50 g/2 oz/¼ cup dairy-free margarine,
plus extra for spreading ⬙**

15 g/½ oz/1 tbsp caster (superfine) sugar

200 ml/7 fl oz/scant 1 cup dairy-free milk ⬙

Jam (conserve) or honey, to serve

1 Line 12 sections of a tartlet tin (patty pan) with paper cake cases (cupcake papers).

2 Sift the flour mix, salt and baking powder together in a bowl.

3 Add the margarine and work in with a fork until the mixture resembles breadcrumbs. Stir in the sugar.

4 Mix with the milk and beat to form a smooth batter.

5 Spoon into the paper cases and bake in a preheated oven at 200°C/400°F/gas mark 6 (fan oven 180°C) for 15 minutes until risen, pale golden and the centres spring back when lightly pressed. Transfer to a wire rack. Serve warm, split and spread with margarine and jam or honey.

Tolerant to ...	Variations
⟍ Wheat	Use plain (all-purpose) flour.
⬙ Dairy	Use ordinary butter or margarine and cows' milk – full-cream for under-5s, semi-skimmed for older children.

Grape Munchies

Make these little crunchy 'cakes' and store them in the fridge for breakfast treats. If your child can't eat corn, use rice crispies instead.

MAKES 6

---

25 g/1 oz/2 tbsp dairy-free margarine 🌢

30 ml/2 tbsp clear honey

75 g/3 oz/ 1½ cups cornflakes

15 g/½ oz/2 tbsp buckwheat grains ☻

Red and green seedless grapes

Dairy-free milk, to serve 🌢

1 Melt the margarine in a saucepan and stir in the honey. Boil for a few seconds.

2 Remove from the heat and add the cornflakes and seeds. Mix until thoroughly coated, then spoon into 12 paper cake cases (cupcake papers). Leave until cold, then store in an airtight container in the fridge.

3 Serve one or two in a bowl, surrounded by whole or halved red and green seedless grapes, with a glass of milk.

Tolerant to ...	Variations
🌢 Dairy	Use butter or other margarine and serve with cows' milk – full-cream for under-5s, semi-skimmed for older children.
☻ Nuts	Use pumpkin or sunflower seeds instead of buckwheat grains (but not for under-5s).

Soft Muesli

Many children, with or without allergies, find traditional Swiss muesli too difficult to chew. This cooked version gives them all the same goodness and flavour, but isn't such hard work! Store it in the fridge in an airtight container.

SERVES 6–8

225 g/8 oz/1 cup brown rice, rinsed

A pinch of salt

75 g/3 oz/1½ cups millet grains

75 g/3 oz/1½ cups buckwheat grains

50 g/2 oz/⅓ cup ready-to-eat dried apricots, chopped

50 g/2 oz/⅓ cup raisins ☺

25 g/1 oz/2 tbsp demerara sugar

Dairy-free milk, to serve ▮

1 Bring a large pan of water to the boil. Add the rice and a pinch of salt, stir well, then cook for 25 minutes. Stir in the buckwheat and millet and continue cooking for about 15 minutes until all the grains are tender, but still have a little 'bite'.

2 Drain, rinse with cold water and drain again. Spread out on kitchen paper (paper towels) and leave to dry and cool.

3 Tip the mixture into a container. Stir in the apricots, raisins and sugar.

4 To serve, spoon into bowls and add milk to taste.

Tolerant to ...	Variations
▮ Dairy	Use cows' milk – full-cream for under-5s, semi-skimmed for older children.
☺ Nuts	Add 45 ml/3 tbsp coconut flakes to the cooked mixture, if liked.

Sausages

SERVES 4

450 g/1 lb belly pork slices

225 g/8 oz bacon pieces

5 ml/1 tsp dried mixed herbs

Freshly ground black pepper

Grilled (broiled) or fried (sautéed) mushrooms or tomatoes and gluten-free tomato ketchup (catsup) or Brown Table Sauce (see page 166), to serve

1 Cut the rind off the belly pork slices and cut out any bones. Cut into chunks. Pick over the bacon, discarding any bones, gristle or rind. Cut into pieces, if necessary.

2 Drop a piece at a time into a food processor with the machine running until finely chopped, or pass through a mincer (grinder).

3 Season with the herbs and pepper.

4 Draw the mixture together into a ball. Remove any white stringy bits of gristly pork fat that haven't been chopped. Shape the mixture into small sausages.

5 Grill on foil on the grill (broiler) rack or dry-fry in a non-stick frying pan (skillet) for about 5–6 minutes, turning occasionally, until cooked through.

6 Serve with mushrooms or tomatoes and ketchup or sauce.

Tolerant to ...	Variations
Wheat	Serve with ordinary ketchup or sauce. For more economical sausages, substitute 100 g/4 oz pork and 50 g/ 2 oz bacon with 175 g/ 6 oz/3 cups fresh breadcrumbs and moisten with a little milk (dairy-free if necessary).

Crispy Hash Browns

SERVES 4

4 large floury potatoes, diced

1 large onion, finely chopped

25 g/1 oz/2 tbsp dairy-free margarine 🥛

Salt and freshly ground black pepper

50 g/2 oz/½ cup wheat-free/gluten-free flour mix ＼

5 ml/1 tsp gluten-free baking powder

120 ml/4 fl oz/½ cup water

Sunflower oil, for cooking

Grilled (broiled) bacon (optional), to serve

1 Boil the potatoes in water for about 5 minutes until just tender. Drain and return to the pan.

2 Meanwhile, fry (sauté) the onion in the margarine in a large frying pan (skillet) for 2 minutes until softened. Add to the potatoes and season lightly. Mash together thoroughly. When cool enough to handle, shape the mixture into eight small, flat, rectangular cakes.

3 Put the flour mix and baking powder in a bowl. Add a pinch of salt. Beat in the water to form a thick batter.

4 Heat enough oil to cover the base of a large frying pan. Dip the cakes in the batter, then fry in the hot oil for 2–3 minutes on each side until crisp and golden brown. Drain on kitchen paper (paper towels). Serve hot with bacon, if liked.

Tolerant to ...	Variations
＼ Wheat	Use plain (all-purpose) flour.
🥛 Dairy	Use butter or ordinary margarine.

SOUPS AND SNACKS

Soups are the ideal way of getting lots of nourishment into your child very easily and this chapter contains some delicious recipes for making your own – including a tomato soup that tastes as near to the canned variety as I could manage! There are also fritters, flavoured potato wedges, pâtés, veggie burgers and a pizza to tempt the taste buds. Many of the recipes would be useful for school lunches (as would some recipes in other sections). Some, like the corn fritters, make a tasty accompaniment to meat or fish as well as being delicious on their own.

CHECK OUT FAST FOODS

Watch out for oven chips (fries) and check the labels carefully. Many of the manufactured ones (those made with processed potato or with added coatings, in particular) will contain wheat flour, casein or other allergens. Those made with pure potato, coated in oil, are fine.

Most canned and packet soups contain either gluten or dairy products. Again, read the labels with care. Pizzas, sandwiches and most snack meals are a problem when you're eating out. If you're going to a café, persuade your child to choose a jacket potato with a suitable topping (such as tuna or crispy bacon). Unfortunately, the fast-food chains are a real problem for most children with allergies. However, they now offer leaflets listing the ingredients in their foods (the information is also available on the internet), so study them in advance to avoid disappointment on arrival!

Creamy Mushroom Soup

I use a food processor to chop the onion and mushrooms but don't process the mushrooms too long, or they will go mushy!

SERVES 4

---

1 small onion, finely chopped

225 g/8 oz button mushrooms, finely chopped

25 g/1 oz/2 tbsp dairy-free margarine 🥛

**600 ml/1 pt/2½ cups vegetable stock, made with
1 dairy-free/gluten-free stock cube**

A good pinch of dried mixed herbs

30 ml/2 tbsp arrowroot

300 ml/½ pt/1¼ cups dairy-free milk 🥛

Salt and freshly ground black pepper

---

1 Cook the onion and mushrooms gently in the margarine for 2 minutes, stirring. Do not allow to brown.

2 Add the stock and herbs. Bring to the boil, reduce the heat, part-cover and simmer gently for 15 minutes.

3 Blend the arrowroot with the milk. Stir into the pan and bring to the boil, stirring until thickened. Do not continue to boil. Season to taste and serve.

Tolerant to ...	Variations
🥛 Dairy	Use only half the quantity of butter or ordinary margarine, then, after thickening, stir in 45 ml/3 tbsp of single (light) cream. Use cows' milk – full-cream for under-5s and semi-skimmed for older children.

Creamy Tomato Soup

SERVES 4

1 small onion, chopped

25 g/1 oz/2 tbsp dairy-free margarine 🖑

400 g/14 oz/1 large can of tomatoes

*300 ml/¹/₂ pt/1¹/₄ cups vegetable stock, made with
1 dairy-free/gluten-free stock cube*

30 ml/2 tbsp tomato purée (paste)

25 ml/1¹/₂ tbsp caster (superfine) sugar

15 ml/1 tbsp arrowroot

150 ml/¹/₄ pt/²/₃ cup dairy-free milk 🖑

Salt and freshly ground black pepper

1 Fry (sauté) the onion in the margarine for 1 minute, stirring occasionally. Reduce the heat to low, cover and sweat the onion for 5 minutes until softened but not browned.

2 Add the tomatoes and break up with a wooden spoon. Stir in the stock, tomato purée and sugar. Bring to the boil, reduce the heat, part-cover and simmer gently for 15 minutes.

3 Purée thoroughly in an electric blender. Blend the arrowroot with the milk in the saucepan. Pour the soup back in the pan and bring to the boil, stirring, until thickened. Do not continue to boil. Season to taste and serve.

Tolerant to ...	Variations
🖑 Dairy	Use only half the quantity of butter or ordinary margarine, then, after thickening, stir in 45 ml/3 tbsp of single (light) cream. Use cows' milk – full-cream for under-5s, semi-skimmed for older children.

Chicken Soup with Rice

My daughter's favourite poem when she was little was 'Chicken Soup with Rice' by Maurice Sendak, so I created this soup specially for her! You can make it with the carcass from the Sunday roast instead of the chicken portion, if you prefer. Also, for a thicker soup, double the quantity of arrowroot.

SERVES 4

---

1 chicken portion

1 small onion, roughly chopped

1 carrot, roughly chopped

1 litre/1³/₄ pts/4¹/₄ cups water

1 dairy-free/gluten-free vegetable stock cube

1 bouquet garni sachet

Salt and freshly ground black pepper

50 g/2 oz/¹/₄ cup long-grain rice

15 ml/1 tbsp arrowroot

300 ml/¹/₂ pt/1¹/₄ cups dairy-free milk

---

1 Put the chicken portion in a large saucepan with the onion, carrot, water, stock cube, bouquet garni sachet and a little salt and pepper.

2 Bring to the boil, reduce the heat, part-cover and simmer gently for 1 hour.

3 Strain the stock into a clean saucepan, pressing the carrot and onions against the sieve (strainer) to extract maximum flavour. Pick all the chicken off the bones, discarding the skin. Cut into small pieces and add to the stock.

4 Add the rice, bring back to the boil, part-cover and simmer for 10 minutes until the rice is tender. Taste and re-season, if necessary.

5 Blend the arrowroot with the milk and stir into the pan. Bring to the boil, stirring until slightly thickened. Do not continue to boil. Serve hot.

Tolerant to ...	Variations
🥛 Dairy	Use cows' milk – full-cream for under-5s, semi-skimmed milk for older children.

Corn Fritters

If your child is allergic to corn, make these with potato flour instead of cornflour and canned or thawed frozen peas instead of the sweetcorn.

MAKES ABOUT 12

---

40 g/1¹/₂ oz/¹/₃ cup rice flour ↖

40 g/1¹/₂ oz/¹/₃ cup cornflour (cornstarch) ↖

A good pinch of salt

15 ml/1 tbsp gluten-free baking powder

105 ml/7 tbsp water

200 g/7 oz/1 small can of sweetcorn (corn), drained

Sunflower oil, for cooking

1 Mix the flours with the salt and baking powder.

2 Stir in the water to form a thick, creamy batter.

3 Stir in the sweetcorn.

4 Heat enough oil to cover the base of a frying pan (skillet). Drop in spoonfuls of the batter. Fry (sauté) until golden underneath. Turn over and cook until crisp. Drain on kitchen paper (paper towels). Serve hot.

Tolerant to ...	Variations
↖ Wheat	Use plain (all-purpose) flour instead of the rice flour and cornflour.

Mixed Vegetable Soup

Many children don't like 'bits' in soup so this smooth soup is an ideal way to give them loads of vegetables without them realising! Ring the changes with other vegetables of your choice.

SERVES 4

---

15 g/½ oz/1 tbsp dairy-free margarine 🔖

1 large potato, cut into small pieces

1 large carrot, sliced

1 leek, well-washed and sliced

1 onion, chopped

¼ small swede (rutabaga), cut into small pieces

1 bay leaf

1 litre/1¾ pts/4¼ cups water or vegetable stock, made with 2 dairy-free/gluten-free stock cubes

15 ml/1 tbsp tomato purée (paste)

Salt and freshly ground black pepper

---

1 Melt the margarine in a large saucepan. Add the vegetables and cook, stirring, for 2 minutes.

2 Add the bay leaf, water or stock and tomato purée. Bring to the boil, part-cover, reduce the heat and simmer gently for 20 minutes or until everything is really tender. Discard the bay leaf.

3 Purée the soup in a blender or food processor and return to the saucepan. Season to taste and reheat if necessary. Serve hot.

Tolerant to ...	Variations
🔖 Dairy	Use butter or ordinary margarine.

Onion Bhajis

These make a delicious spicy snack.

SERVES 4

75 g/3 oz/³⁄₄ cup gram flour

60 ml/4 tbsp water

2.5 ml/¹⁄₂ tsp chilli powder

1.5 ml/¹⁄₄ tsp ground turmeric

5 ml/1 tsp ground coriander (cilantro)

5 ml/1 tsp salt

Sunflower oil, for cooking

15 ml/1 tbsp chopped fresh coriander

2 onions, quartered and thinly sliced

1 Mix the flour with the water to make a thick, creamy batter.

2 Mix in the spices and salt and beat until smooth. Leave to stand for 30 minutes.

3 Heat about 1 cm/¹⁄₂ in of oil in a large frying pan (skillet) until a cornflake dropped in rises to the surface and sizzles immediately.

4 Meanwhile, mix the coriander and onion into the batter. Drop spoonfuls of the mixture into the hot oil and cook for about 5 minutes until golden, turning once. Drain on kitchen paper (paper towels).

5 Serve hot or cold.

Potato Wedges with Pepper Dip

These use no fat, which makes them nutritious for all the family! For crisp wedges, cut the potatoes fairly thinly, for soft-centred ones, cut them thicker. If your child is allergic to tomatoes, omit the ketchup. For a spicy version, add a few drops of Tabasco to the dip.

SERVES 4

---

450 g/1 lb potatoes, scrubbed

45 ml/3 tbsp dairy-free milk 🗋

5 ml/1 tsp paprika

5 ml/1 tsp garlic salt

Freshly ground black pepper

For the dip:

200 g/7 oz/1 small can of pimientos, drained

2 spring onions (scallions), trimmed and cut into short lengths

5 ml/1 tsp clear honey

15 ml/1 tbsp gluten-free tomato ketchup (catsup)

---

1 Cut the potatoes into halves, then into wedges.

2 Put the milk in a bowl. Add the potatoes and stir to coat.

3 Mix the paprika, garlic salt and a good grinding of pepper together.

4 Arrange the wet potato wedges on a non-stick baking (cookie) sheet. Sprinkle with half the paprika mixture. Turn the wedges over and sprinkle the other sides.

5 Bake towards the top of a preheated oven at 200°C/ 400°F/gas mark 6 (fan oven 180°C) for about 25 minutes, turning over halfway through cooking, until crisp and deep golden brown (take care with thin-cut ones, as they burn quickly).

6 Put all the ingredients for the dip in a blender or food processor and run the machine until well blended. Tip into a small bowl and serve with the wedges.

Tolerant to ...	Variations
🥄 Dairy	Use cows' milk – full-cream for under-5s, semi-skimmed milk for older children.

Quick-cook Pâté

Use this as a spread on bread, rice cakes or crackers.

SERVES 6–8
---

100 g/4 oz/¹/₂ cup dairy-free margarine 🥄

225 g/8 oz chicken livers, trimmed and roughly chopped

50 g/2 oz streaky bacon, rinded and diced

1 garlic clove, crushed, or ¹/₂ small onion, finely chopped

2.5 ml/¹/₂ tsp dried mixed herbs

15 ml/1 tbsp apple juice

Salt and freshly ground black pepper

1 Melt half the margarine in a saucepan. Add all the remaining ingredients and cook, stirring, for 6 minutes until the chicken livers are just cooked but still pink – don't overcook or they will go hard.

2 Purée in a blender or food processor.

3 Turn into a small container with a lid and leave to cool. Melt the remaining margarine and pour over, then chill until fairly firm. Use as required.

Tolerant to ...	Variations
🥄 Dairy	Use butter or ordinary margarine.

Veggie Burgers

MAKES 8

1 small potato, cut into small pieces

1 small parsnip, cut into small pieces

1 small carrot, cut into small pieces

15 g/½ oz/1 tbsp dairy-free margarine ❦

225 g/8 oz/1 small can of butter (lima) beans, drained

Salt and freshly ground black pepper

25 g/1 oz/¼ cup thawed frozen peas

15 ml/1 tbsp potato flour

45 ml/3 tbsp dairy-free milk ❦ ⌒

100 g/4 oz plain potato crisps (chips), crushed

A little sunflower oil

Fresh Tomato Salsa (see page 170) or rounds of wheat-free/gluten-free bread and gluten-free tomato ketchup (catsup), to serve ❖

1 Boil the potato, parsnip and carrot together in water until really tender. Drain and return to the pan. Heat gently, stirring, to dry out. Mash with the margarine, butter beans and some salt and pepper.

2 Stir in the peas and flour.

3 Shape into eight small cakes. Dip in the milk, then the crushed crisps to coat completely, pressing them gently into the surface. Chill for at least 30 minutes, if possible.

4 Brush a piece of foil on a grill (broiler) rack with a little oil. Add the burgers and brush lightly with oil. Grill (broil) for about 4 minutes on each side until golden and crisp. Serve hot or cold with Fresh Tomato Salsa or sandwich each one between two rounds of wheat-free/gluten-free bread, with a little ketchup added.

Tolerant to ...	Variations
♥ Dairy	Use butter or ordinary margarine. Use cows' milk – full-cream for under-5s, semi-skimmed for older children.
↶ Eggs	Use 1 beaten egg instead of the milk, if liked.
↖ Wheat	Serve in bread rolls.

Vegetable Pâté

SERVES 4–6

15 g/¹/₂ oz/1 tbsp dairy-free margarine ♥

1 onion, chopped

1 courgette (zucchini), chopped

1 carrot, chopped

425 g/15 oz/1 large can of red kidney beans, drained

5 ml/1 tsp lemon juice

5 ml/1 tsp Marmite or other yeast extract

15 ml/1 tbsp chopped fresh parsley

Salt and freshly ground black pepper

1 Melt the margarine in a saucepan. Add the onion, courgette and carrot and cook, stirring, for 2 minutes. Cover with a lid and cook over a gentle heat for about 6 minutes until tender.

2 Tip the mixture into a blender or food processor. Add all the remaining ingredients except the salt and pepper and purée until smooth. Season to taste.

3 Tip into a container. Cool, then store in the fridge.

Tolerant to ...	Variations
♥ Dairy	Use butter or ordinary margarine.

Cheese and Tomato Pizza

If your child can't eat tomatoes, use puréed, well-drained canned carrots or pimientos instead. You can add other toppings of your choice, such as olives, mushrooms, etc., before baking, and you can also use soya, goats' or sheep's cheese if your child can tolerate them. If you make up the whole soft bread quantity, you can make two pizzas and freeze one for another day.

SERVES 2 OR 4

---

*½ quantity of **Wheat-free/Gluten-free Soft White Bread** dough (see page 122)* ╲

....

30 ml/2 tbsp tomato purée (paste)

....

1.5 ml/¼ tsp dried oregano

....

*50 g/2 oz/½ cup grated **No-allergen Hard Cheese** (see page 178)* 🥄

....

1 Make up the dough and use a wet knife or the back of a spoon to spread it out to a 20 cm/8 in round on an oiled baking (cookie) sheet. The dough will slide about a bit on the oil but persevere! Leave in a warm place for 30 minutes to rise slightly.

2 Bake in a preheated oven at 200°C/400°F/gas mark 6 (fan oven 180°C) for 10 minutes.

3 Spread with the tomato purée, then sprinkle with the oregano and cheese. Return to the oven for about 6 minutes or until golden and crisp round the edges and the cheese has melted. Serve hot, cut into wedges.

Tolerant to ...	Variations
╲ Wheat	Use your usual pizza base recipe.
🥄 Dairy	Use Cheddar or other hard cheese.

MEAT AND POULTRY MAIN MEALS

There is no point in my giving you meat-and-two-veg-type recipes as they are all easy to prepare and quite acceptable whatever allergies your child has. Instead, for this chapter I've created great versions of favourite junior foods – including chicken nuggets and beefburgers – with lots of tasty recipes for family meals that would normally have eggs, dairy products, wheat or gluten in them. I am sure the whole family will enjoy the recipes so you won't have to make special dishes all the time from now on.

PASTA AND NOODLES

Chinese rice noodles and Japanese buckwheat noodles, which my family like better than specialist corn pasta as an alternative to wheat varieties, are widely available in supermarkets. If I buy pasta shapes, I buy rice ones too, as we think they have a more pleasant texture than corn pasta, but the choice is yours! For lasagne, I make home-made buckwheat pasta – see my simple recipe on page 72 – and you'll find a recipe for ravioli on page 98.

Country Hot Pot

You can use cooked, leftover vegetables in this dish.

SERVES 4

---

1 onion, chopped

225 g/8 oz minced (ground) beef or lamb

350 g/12 oz frozen mixed country vegetables

*300 ml/¹/₂ pt/1¹/₄ cups vegetable stock, made with
1 dairy-free/gluten-free stock cube*

450 g/1 lb potatoes, scrubbed and sliced

15 ml/1 tbsp potato flour

30 ml/2 tbsp water

400 g/14 oz/1 large can of gluten-free baked beans

5 ml/1 tsp yeast extract (optional)

Salt and freshly ground black pepper

15 g/¹/₂ oz/1 tbsp dairy-free margarine

Broccoli, to serve

1 Put the onion and mince in a flameproof casserole (Dutch oven) and cook, stirring, until all the grains of meat are separate and no longer pink.

2 Add the country vegetables and stock and cook for 10 minutes until just tender.

3 Meanwhile, boil the potatoes in a separate pan of lightly salted water until tender. Drain.

4 Blend the potato flour with the measured water and stir into the meat and vegetables. Bring to the boil and cook for 1 minute, stirring. Stir in the beans and yeast extract. Season to taste.

5 Arrange the sliced potatoes over the top. Dot the margarine over the surface. Place under a preheated grill (broiler) for about 4 minutes until turning golden on top. Serve hot with broccoli.

Tolerant to ...	Variations
Wheat	Use plain (all-purpose) flour.
Dairy	Use butter or ordinary margarine.

Beefburgers

Use minced lamb, pork, chicken or turkey, if you prefer. You can buy a burger press quite cheaply, otherwise use a small, clean 225 g/8 oz food can to mould the burgers (see method). If your child likes cheeseburgers, use soya or rice cheese slices, or cut thin slices of No-allergen Hard Cheese (see page 178).

SERVES 4

225g/8 oz lean minced (ground) beef

5 ml/1 tsp dried minced onion

5 ml/1 tsp dried mixed herbs

Salt and freshly ground black pepper

15 ml/1 tbsp potato flour

A little sunflower oil

*8 fairly thick slices of wheat-free/gluten-free bread
(preferably the milk bread on page 120)*

Gluten-free tomato ketchup (catsup)

4 Dill-pickled Cucumber Slices (see page 169)

1 small onion, finely chopped

A little shredded lettuce

1 Mix the minced meat with the dried onion, herbs, a little salt and pepper and the potato flour.

2 Divide the mixture into four portions. Cut eight circles of non-stick baking parchment the size of your burger press (unless your press comes complete with the paper discs) or 'can' cutter.

3 If using a press, follow the manufacturer's instructions. If using a can, place it on a board. Put one paper disc in the can. Add one portion of the meat mixture. Place another disc of paper on top. Lay the can lid on top. Place a smaller can on top for added leverage, then press down firmly with your hands to flatten the mixture. You can then remove the burger, sandwiched between two discs of non-stick baking parchment, from the can. Repeat with the remainder.

4 Place on foil on a grill (broiler) rack and brush with a little oil. Grill (broil) for about 3–4 minutes on each side until golden brown and cooked through.

5 Cut the largest rounds possible from the bread slices, using a biscuit (cookie) cutter. (Use the crusts for crumbs for a separate recipe.)

6 Spread four slices with a little ketchup and top with a burger. Top each burger with a Dill-pickled Cucumber Slice, a little chopped onion and shredded lettuce. Top with the second slices of bread and serve.

Tolerant to ...	Variations
Wheat	Use soft, white rolls instead of the wheat-free/gluten-free bread. If your child can tolerate gluten, use bought dill pickles.
Eggs	Use a small beaten egg instead of potato flour to bind the mixture.

Rocky Ribs

If your child is allergic to tomatoes, use my Brown Table Sauce (see page 166) instead of the tomato ketchup. If you can't find gluten-free Worcestershire sauce, use balsamic vinegar, a few drops of Tabasco sauce and a good pinch of salt.

SERVES 4

---

900 g/2 lb Chinese pork spare ribs

75 ml/5 tbsp white wine vinegar

1 garlic clove, crushed

60 ml/4 tbsp clear honey

60 ml/4 tbsp gluten-free tomato ketchup (catsup)

45 ml/3 tbsp gluten-free Worcestershire sauce ࿇

5 ml/1 tsp gluten-free English mustard

---

1 Put the ribs in a large saucepan. Cover with water and add half the vinegar. Bring to the boil, reduce the heat, cover and simmer for 1 hour. Drain and place in a single layer in a roasting tin (pan).

2 Mix all the other ingredients together, including the remaining vinegar. Pour over the meat and turn each piece to coat completely.

3 Bake in a preheated oven at 200°C/400°F/gas mark 6 (fan oven 180°C) for about 35 minutes until richly coated in the sticky sauce. Serve hot.

Tolerant to ...	Variations
࿇ Soya	Use soy sauce (gluten-free if necessary) instead of the Worcestershire sauce.

Mini Toad-in-the-hole

Remember that xanthum gum contains corn, so if your child can't tolerate it, use guar gum instead.

SERVES 4

¼ quantity of sausagemeat (see page 51)

70 g/2¾ oz/scant ¾ cup wheat-free/gluten-free flour mix, plus extra for dusting ❧

30 ml/2 tbsp sunflower oil, for cooking

3 g/rounded ½ tsp xanthum gum ❧

10 ml/2 tsp gluten-free baking powder

A pinch of salt

50 g/2 oz grated potato ⬭

100 ml/3½ fl oz/scant ½ cup dairy-free milk 🥛

100 ml/3½ fl oz/scant ½ cup water

Wheat-free/gluten-free gravy (see page 176), ❧
potatoes, carrots and broccoli, to serve

---

1 Shape the sausagemeat into 36 very small balls, with hands lightly dusted with wheat-free/gluten-free flour mix.

2 Divide among the 12 sections of a tartlet tin (patty pan) and add about 2.5 ml/½ tsp of oil to each.

3 Put the tin towards the top of a preheated oven at 200°C/400°F/gas mark 6 (fan oven 180°C) for about 5 minutes until sizzling.

4 Meanwhile, mix the flour, gum, baking powder and salt in a bowl. Add the potato and half the milk and water and beat until smooth. Stir in the remaining milk and water and mix well.

5 When the sausages are sizzling, spoon in the batter. Cook for 25 minutes until risen, crisp and golden. Remove from the tin and serve hot with gravy, potatoes, carrots and broccoli.

Tolerant to ...	Variations
⟍ Wheat	Use plain (all-purpose flour), omitting the gum, and ordinary gravy.
🥛 Dairy	Use cows' milk – full-cream for under-5s, semi-skimmed for older children.
⌣ Eggs	Use 1 small egg, beaten, instead of the potato.

Baked Lasagne

If your child is allergic to tomatoes, use a large can of pimientos or carrots, drained and puréed, instead of the tomatoes and omit the tomato purée and sugar. If your child is allergic to corn, use rice flour for dusting.

SERVES 4

For the buckwheat pasta:

50 g/2 oz/½ cup buckwheat flour

25 g/1 oz/¼ cup potato flour

A good pinch of salt

7.5 ml/1½ tsp No Egg egg replacer (see page 20) ☺

60 ml/4 tbsp warm water

A little cornflour (cornstarch), for dusting

For the sauce:

1 onion, finely chopped

1 garlic clove, crushed

1 carrot, finely chopped

350 g/12 oz minced (ground) beef or lamb

400 g/14 oz/1 large can of chopped tomatoes

15 ml/1 tbsp tomato purée (paste)

5 ml/1 tsp caster (superfine) sugar

Salt and freshly ground black pepper

5 ml/1 tsp dried oregano

For the topping:

1½ quantities of Cheese Sauce (see page 174) 🌿

A green salad, to serve

1 Mix the flours together with the salt in a bowl.

2 Whisk the egg replacer and water together until frothy and work with a fork into the flours until a dough is forming, then knead together with your hands. Turn out on to a board and knead until fairly smooth. Wrap in clingfilm (plastic wrap) and leave to rest for 15 minutes.

3 Roll out very thinly on a board dusted with cornflour. Cut into six strips about 7.5 × 15 cm/3 × 6 in, re-kneading and rolling the trimmings as necessary. Leave to dry on the board while you prepare the sauce.

4 Put the onion, garlic, carrot and meat in a saucepan and dry-fry, stirring, until all the grains of meat are separate and no longer pink.

5 Add the tomatoes, purée, sugar, a very little salt, some pepper and the oregano. Bring to the boil, stirring, reduce the heat and simmer for 15 minutes.

6 Put a spoonful of the meat sauce in the base of a shallow 1.2 litre/2 pt/5 cup ovenproof dish. Top with two strips of lasagne. Layer half the remaining meat, two more strips of pasta, then the remaining meat and the last two strips of pasta. Cover with the cheese sauce.

7 Bake in a preheated oven at 190°C/375°F/gas mark 5 (fan oven 170°C) for about 35 minutes until golden and cooked through. Serve hot with a green salad.

Tolerant to ...	Variations
⬩ Wheat	Use wholemeal or plain (all-purpose) flour instead of the buckwheat.
⬩ Eggs	Use 1 large beaten egg instead of the egg replacer and warm water. You may need to add a little water to the dough – especially if you use wheat flour.
⬩ Dairy	Make the sauce to your usual recipe, using cows' milk – full-cream for under-5s, semi-skimmed for older children – and grated Cheddar cheese.

Quinoa Couscous

SERVES 4

---

1 bunch of spring onions (scallions), chopped

250 g/9 oz lamb neck fillets, trimmed and cut into small pieces

1 large courgette (zucchini), cut into small chunks

15 g/¹/₂ oz/1 tbsp dairy-free margarine 🦪

2.5 ml/¹/₂ tsp ground cumin

2.5 ml/¹/₂ tsp ground cinnamon

50 g/2 oz/¹/₃ cup ready-to-eat dried apricots, chopped

100 g/4 oz/1 cup quinoa, rinsed ✎

750 ml/ 1¹/₄ pts/3 cups vegetable stock, made with 1 dairy-free/gluten-free stock cube

Salt and freshly ground black pepper

A little chopped fresh parsley, mint or coriander (cilantro), for garnishing

---

1 In a large frying pan (skillet), fry (sauté) the lamb, spring onions and courgette in the margarine for 2 minutes, stirring occasionally. Stir in the spices.

2 Stir in the apricots, quinoa and stock. Bring to the boil, stir, reduce the heat slightly and simmer fairly rapidly for 20 minutes or until the meat is tender and the quinoa has absorbed the liquid, stirring occasionally.

3 Season to taste and serve garnished with a little chopped parsley, mint or coriander.

Tolerant to ...	Variations
✎ Wheat	Use couscous instead of quinoa.
🦪 Dairy	Use butter or ordinary margarine.

Chinese Chicken Drumsticks

If you don't have gluten-free Worcestershire sauce, use my Brown Table Sauce (see page 166) or balsamic vinegar, a few drops of Tabasco sauce and a pinch of salt instead. This quantity will also coat 24 chicken wings (not whole portions).

MAKES 10

15 ml/1 tbsp white wine vinegar

45 ml/3 tbsp sunflower oil

15 ml/1 tbsp gluten-free Worcestershire sauce

2.5 ml/½ tsp Marmite or other yeast extract

25 ml/1½ tbsp clear honey

25 ml/1½ tbsp plum jam (conserve)

2.5 ml/½ tsp Chinese five-spice powder

10 small chicken drumsticks

1 Mix all the ingredients except the chicken together in a large roasting tin (pan) until well blended.

2 Add the chicken drumsticks and turn to coat completely. Cover and leave to marinate for 1 hour.

3 Uncover and bake in a preheated oven at 180°C/ 350°F/gas mark 4 (fan oven 160°C) for about 50 minutes to 1 hour, turning once or twice during cooking, until tender and coated in a sticky glaze.

4 Serve hot or cold.

Crunchy Turkey Slices

Try these with pork steaks too.

SERVES 4

---

4 turkey breast steaks

75 g/3 oz/³⁄₄ cup millet flakes ✎

15 ml/1 tbsp dried minced (ground) onion ✎

5 ml/1 tsp dried sage ✎

Salt and freshly ground black pepper

45 ml/3 tbsp dairy-free milk 🗑 ⌒

Sunflower oil, for cooking

Wedges of lemon and sprigs of fresh parsley, for garnishing

Creamed potatoes and French (green) beans, to serve

---

1 Put the turkey steaks one at a time in a plastic bag and beat with a rolling pin or meat mallet until flattened.

2 Mix the millet with the dried onion, herbs and a little salt and pepper.

3 Dip each steak first in milk, then in the millet mixture, to coat completely.

4 Heat the oil in a large frying pan (skillet) and fry (sauté) the turkey steaks for about 3 minutes on each side until golden brown and cooked through. Drain on kitchen paper (paper towels).

5 Transfer to warm plates, garnish with lemon wedges and sprigs of parsley and serve hot with creamed potatoes and French beans.

Tolerant to ...	Variations
Wheat	Use fresh breadcrumbs instead of the millet flakes, or substitute a packet of stuffing mix instead of the flakes, onion and herbs.
Dairy	Use cows' milk – full-cream for under-5s, semi-skimmed for older children.
Eggs	Use 1 large beaten egg instead of the milk for coating the steaks, if preferred.

Sunny Rice Supper

SERVES 4

175 g/6 oz/³/₄ cup long-grain rice

50 g/2 oz/¹/₂ cup frozen peas

5 cm/2 in piece of cucumber, diced

175 g/6 oz cooked chicken, diced

225 g/8 oz/1 small can of pineapple pieces, drained, reserving the juice

60 ml/4 tbsp Egg-free Mayonnaise (see page 177) ⏺

Salt and freshly ground black pepper

A few lettuce leaves

1 Cook the rice in plenty of boiling, lightly salted water for 5 minutes. Add the peas and cook for a further 5 minutes until just tender. Drain, rinse with cold water and drain again.

2 Place in a bowl and add the cucumber, chicken and pineapple.

3 Thin the mayonnaise with about 15 ml/1 tbsp of the pineapple juice. Fold into the rice mixture. Season to taste.

4 Pile on to lettuce leaves and serve.

Tolerant to ...	Variations
⏺ Eggs	Use ordinary mayonnaise.

Chinese Noodle Doodles

If your child can't tolerate soya, use balsamic vinegar instead of soy sauce and season well with salt. Add extra vegetables, such as thin strips of celery, sliced mushrooms or wedges of tomato, if your child likes them.

SERVES 4

250 g/9 oz rice noodles

1 carrot, cut into thin matchsticks

1 bunch of spring onions (scallions), cut into short lengths

1 red (bell) pepper, cut into thin strips

30 ml/2 tbsp sunflower oil

350 g/12 oz turkey, chicken, beef or pork stir-fry meat

1 large courgette (zucchini), cut into thin matchsticks

5 cm/2 in piece of cucumber, cut into thin matchsticks

90 ml/6 tbsp apple juice

45 ml/3 tbsp gluten-free soy sauce

Freshly ground black pepper

1 Put the noodles in a bowl. Cover with boiling water and leave to stand while you cook the stir-fry.

2 Meanwhile, stir-fry the carrot, spring onions and pepper in the oil for 2 minutes, stirring.

3 Add the meat and stir-fry for 3 minutes.

4 Add the courgette and cucumber and stir-fry for a further 2 minutes.

5 Add all the remaining ingredients except the noodles and cook, stirring, for 1 minute.

6 Drain the noodles. Spoon them into warm bowls. Top with the stir-fry and serve straight away.

Mini Kievs

I use chicken breasts and mince them myself but you can buy ready-minced chicken if you prefer.

SERVES 4

---

50 g/2 oz/¼ cup dairy-free margarine 🥛

1 small garlic clove, crushed

2.5 ml/½ tsp dried mixed herbs

Salt and freshly ground black pepper

350 g/12 oz minced (ground) chicken

10 ml/2 tsp potato flour

5 ml/1 tsp paprika

30 ml/2 tbsp rice flour 🌾

45 ml/3 tbsp dairy-free milk 🥛 🌀

50 g/2 oz/1 cup wheat-free/gluten-free breadcrumbs 🌾

Sunflower oil, for shallow-frying

Rice, carrots and broccoli, to serve

---

1 Mash the margarine with the garlic, herbs and a little salt and pepper. Shape into a roll on a piece of greaseproof (waxed) paper and roll up in the paper. Freeze until firm.

2 Mix the minced chicken with the potato flour, a little salt and pepper and the paprika. Mix well and divide into 12 pieces.

3 Cut the frozen garlic 'butter' into 12 pieces. Flatten each piece of mince and put a piece of the butter in the centre. Shape into a ball around the butter and roll in the rice flour. Coat in milk, then the breadcrumbs to cover thoroughly. Chill, if time allows, before cooking.

4 Heat about 5 mm/¼ in of oil in a large frying pan (skillet). Shallow-fry the balls for about 6 minutes, turning once or twice, until golden brown and cooked through. Drain on kitchen paper (paper towels) and serve straight away with rice, carrots and broccoli.

Tolerant to ...	Variations
Dairy	Use butter or ordinary margarine and cows' milk – full-cream for under-5s, semi-skimmed for older children.
Eggs	Use 1 beaten egg instead of milk to coat the chicken, if you prefer.
Wheat	Use plain (all-purpose) flour instead of the rice flour, and use ordinary breadcrumbs.

Chicken Nuggets

Serve the Potato Wedges plain, without their dip.

SERVES 4

3–4 skinless chicken breasts, cut into bite-sized chunks

30 ml/2 tbsp rice flour ✎

Salt and freshly ground black pepper

50 g/2 oz plain potato crisps (chips), fairly finely crushed

5 ml/1 tsp paprika

60 ml/4 tbsp dairy-free milk 🥛 ⌾

Sunflower oil, for cooking

Barbecue Dipping Sauce (see page 167), Potato Wedges (see page 60) and peas, to serve

---

1 Toss the chicken in the rice flour, seasoned with a little salt and pepper.

2 Mix the crisps with the paprika on a plate. Put the milk in a shallow dish.

3 Dip the chicken in the milk, then the crisps, until well coated. If necessary, repeat the process.

4 Heat just enough oil to cover the base of a frying pan (skillet). Add the chicken and fry (sauté) for about 2–3 minutes on each side until golden and cooked through. Drain on kitchen paper (paper towels), serve with Barbecue Dipping Sauce, Potato Wedges and peas.

Tolerant to ...	Variations
✎ Wheat	Use plain (all-purpose) flour and breadcrumbs instead of crisps, if liked.
🥛 Dairy	Use cows' milk – full-cream for under-5s, semi-skimmed for older children.
⌾ Eggs	Use 1 beaten egg instead of the milk, if preferred, for coating the chicken.

SEAFOOD AND VEGETABLE MAIN MEALS

Fish is a potential allergen in older children, but it is a highly nutritious food so I have included it here. Not only does it provide easily digestible protein, but also vitamins A and D, plus essential omega 3 fatty acids, which can help prevent heart disease in later life. Many popular ready-made fish dishes for children are full of allergens, such as crumb coatings and egg batters, but for this chapter I've created all their favourites – and many more too – without an allergen in sight. You will also find a few vegetarian main meals, all nutritionally balanced and designed specifically to appeal to children of all ages (and most adults too!).

CANS FOR CONVENIENCE AND GOODNESS

Canned fish, such as tuna, sardines, pilchards, mackerel and salmon, make delicious sandwiches and other snack meals. Try sardines, lightly grilled (broiled), on fingers of toast (wheat-fee/gluten-free, if necessary), or tuna flaked in a salad with cold new potatoes, French (green) beans and a little oil and wine vinegar. Encourage your children to eat the soft bones in canned fish, too, as they are a great source of calcium (if you mash them up with the fish, they'll never notice).

Salmon Fish Cakes

These are also tasty made with tuna and flavoured with chopped fresh parsley instead of the chives.

SERVES 4

---

2 potatoes, scrubbed

A knob of dairy-free margarine 🌱

200 g/7 oz/1 small can of salmon, drained

15 ml/1 tbsp snipped fresh chives

Salt and freshly ground black pepper

2.5 ml/½ tsp lemon juice (optional)

45 ml/3 tbsp potato flour

45 ml/3 tbsp dairy-free milk 🌱 ⬭

50 g/2 oz/½ cup millet flakes ➘

Sunflower oil, for shallow-frying

Peas, to serve

---

1 Prick the potatoes all over and cook in the microwave for 7–8 minutes until soft, then remove the skins. Alternatively, peel and cut them into chunks and cook them in boiling water until tender, then drain well. Mash with the margarine.

2 Remove any skin from the fish. Discard the bones, if liked, but, ideally, mash them thoroughly with the fish. Stir the fish into the potatoes and add the chives, a little salt and pepper and lemon juice, if using.

3 Shape the mixture into four fish-shaped cakes, about 2 cm/¾ in thick. Dip the cakes in the potato flour, then in the milk, then the millet flakes to coat completely. Chill for 30 minutes.

4 Shallow-fry the cakes in hot oil for about 2 minutes on each side, until golden brown. Drain on kitchen paper (paper towels). Alternatively, brush lightly with oil and place on lightly oiled foil on a grill (broiler) rack and grill (broil) for 4–5 minutes on each side until golden brown and hot through.

5 Transfer the fish cakes to warm plates and serve with peas.

Tolerant to ...	Variations
Eggs	Use 1 beaten egg to coat the fish cakes instead of the milk, if liked.
Dairy	Use butter or ordinary margarine and cows' milk – full-cream for under-5s, semi-skimmed for older children.
Wheat	Use plain (all-purpose) flour instead of the potato flour and dried breadcrumbs instead of the millet flakes.

Tuna and Broccoli Pasta

If your child is allergic to corn, use potato flour instead of cornflour. You can use hard sheep's, goats' or soya cheese if your child can tolerate them.

SERVES 4

225 g/8 oz wheat-free/gluten-free pasta shapes ➘

175 g/6 oz broccoli, cut into tiny florets

20 g/³⁄₄ oz/3 tbsp cornflour (cornstarch)

300 ml/¹⁄₂ pt/1¹⁄₄ cups dairy-free milk 🖒

15 g/¹⁄₂ oz/1 tbsp dairy-free margarine 🖒

185 g/6¹⁄₂ oz/1 small can of tuna, drained

5 ml/1 tsp lemon juice (optional)

2.5 ml/¹⁄₂ tsp dried oregano

Salt and freshly ground black pepper

100 g/4 oz streaky bacon, rinded and diced (optional)

50 g/2 oz/¹⁄₂ cup grated No-allergen Hard Cheese (see page 178), to serve 🖒

---

1 Cook the pasta according to the packet directions, adding the broccoli for the last 5 minutes' cooking time. Drain and return to the pan.

2 Meanwhile, blend the cornflour with a little of the milk in a separate saucepan. Stir in the remaining milk and add the margarine. Bring to the boil and cook, stirring, for 1 minute until thickened.

3 Stir in the tuna, lemon juice, if using, oregano and a little salt and pepper.

4 Tip this mixture into the pasta and broccoli and toss gently over a low heat until well mixed.

5 If using bacon, quickly dry-fry until crisp. Drain on
   kitchen paper (paper towels). Spoon the pasta into
   warm bowls, sprinkle with the cheese and bacon, if
   using, and serve hot.

Tolerant to ...	Variations
Wheat	Use ordinary pasta.
Dairy	Use cows' milk – full-cream for under-5s, semi-skimmed for older children – butter or ordinary margarine and Cheddar cheese.

Fish and Chips

If your child can't tolerate corn, use potato flour instead of cornflour.

SERVES 4

---

4 good-sized potatoes, scrubbed or peeled

Sunflower oil, for shallow-frying

For the fritter batter:

40 g/1½ oz/⅓ cup cornflour (cornstarch)

40 g/1½ oz/⅓ cup rice flour

A good pinch of salt

15 ml/1 tbsp gluten-free baking powder

105 ml/7 tbsp water

4 small fillets of cod or haddock, skinned

Peas and gluten-free tomato ketchup (catsup), to serve

1 Cut the potatoes into thick slices, then cut each slice into fingers. Place in a bowl of cold water and soak for at least 5 minutes. Drain and dry on kitchen paper (paper towels).

2 Heat about 2.5 cm/1 in sunflower oil in a large frying pan (skillet). Lower the chips (fries) carefully into the oil (I slide them down a fish slice held against the side of the pan to prevent splashing).

3 Cook the chips for about 8 minutes, turning once or twice, until crisp and golden. Drain on kitchen paper.

4 Meanwhile, mix the flours with the salt and baking powder and stir in enough water to form a thick, creamy batter.

5 Pour oil to a depth of about 5 mm/^{1}/$_4$ in into another pan and heat. Dip the fish in the batter and add to the pan. Cook for about 3 minutes on each side until crisp, golden and cooked through. Drain on kitchen paper.

6 Transfer to warm plates and serve with peas and tomato ketchup.

Tolerant to ...	Variations
Wheat	Use plain (all-purpose) flour instead of the rice flour and cornflour.

Crinkly Fish Sticks with Pea Dip

*For Traditional-style Fish Fingers, make the coating with
breadcrumbs (wheat-free/gluten-free if necessary) mixed with
2.5 ml/½ tsp each of paprika and turmeric and a little salt
and pepper.*

SERVES 4

---

450 g/1 lb thick white fish fillet, skinned

100 g/4 oz plain potato crisps (chips), crushed

30 ml/2 tbsp dried minced (ground) onion

50 g/2 oz/½ cup potato flour ✎

75 ml/5 tbsp dairy-free milk 🥛

300 g/11 oz/1 medium can of garden peas

Sunflower oil, for shallow-frying

Baby new potatoes and carrots, to serve

1 Cut the fish into chunky fingers. Mix the crisps with
   the dried onion on a plate. Dip the fish sticks in the
   flour, then the milk, then the crisp mixture to coat
   completely. Chill until ready to cook.

2 Purée the peas in a blender or food processor with a
   little of their liquid to form a thick, dipping sauce. Tip
   into a small saucepan and heat through.

3 Pour oil to a depth of 5 mm/¼ in into a large frying
   pan (skillet). Heat, then fry (sauté) the fish for 3
   minutes on each side until crisp and golden brown.
   Drain on kitchen paper (paper towels).

4 Serve with baby new potatoes and carrots and the pea
   sauce in small bowls to one side.

Tolerant to ...	Variations
✎ Wheat	Use plain (all-purpose) flour.
🥛 Dairy	Use cows' milk – full-cream for under-5s, semi-skimmed for older children.

Fish and Rootie Wedges

SERVES 4

2 large potatoes, scrubbed and grated

1 large carrot, grated

¼ small swede (rutabaga), grated

Salt and freshly ground black pepper

15 g/½ oz/1 tbsp dairy-free margarine 🛇

30 ml/2 tbsp sunflower oil

450 g/1 lb white fish fillet, skinned and cubed

Gluten-free tomato ketchup (catsup) or Brown Table Sauce (see page 166) and French (green) beans, to serve

1 Mix the grated vegetables together and squeeze thoroughly to remove excess moisture. Season lightly.

2 Heat the margarine and oil in a large frying pan (skillet). Add half the vegetable mixture and press down well. Cover with the cubes of fish, then the remaining vegetable mixture, again, pressing down well. Cover with a lid or foil and cook over a fairly gentle heat for about 30 minutes or until cooked through.

3 Turn the fish and potato cake out on to a warm plate, browned side up. Cut into wedges. Transfer to warm plates and serve with ketchup or brown sauce and French beans.

Tolerant to ...	Variations
🛇 Dairy	Use butter or ordinary margarine.

Broad Bean Risotto

You can use hard sheep's, goats' or soya cheese, if your child can tolerate them.

SERVES 4

250 g/9 oz shelled fresh or frozen broad (fava) beans

Salt and freshly ground black pepper

25 g/1 oz/2 tbsp dairy-free margarine 🍶

1 bunch of spring onions (scallions), chopped

225 g/8 oz/1 cup round-grain (pudding) rice

900 ml/1½ pts/3¾ cups hot vegetable stock, made with 2 dairy-free/gluten-free vegetable stock cubes

50 g/2 oz/¼ cup grated No-allergen Hard Cheese (see page 178) 🍶

15 ml/1 tbsp chopped fresh parsley

1   Cook the broad beans in lightly salted boiling water for 5 minutes until tender. Drain and remove the skins, if liked.

2   Melt the margarine in a large saucepan. Add the spring onions and cook, stirring, for 2 minutes. Stir in the rice until every grain is glistening.

3   Pour on about a quarter of the hot stock, bring to the boil, reduce the heat and simmer until the stock is absorbed. Repeat with a little more stock at a time until the rice is just tender but still has some 'bite', and all the liquid is used. The risotto should be creamy.

4   Stir in the broad beans and cheese and season to taste. Serve sprinkled with the parsley.

Tolerant to ...	Variations
🍶 Dairy	Use butter or ordinary margarine and Parmesan or Cheddar cheese.

Mariner's Pizza

You can also use hard sheep's cheese, goats' cheese, buffalo Mozzarella or soya cheese, depending on your child's allergies. This recipe contains xanthum gum, which is not suitable if your child is allergic to corn – use guar gum instead.

SERVES 4

---

225 g/8 oz/2 cups Wheat-free/Gluten-free Flour Mix (see page 164), plus extra for dusting ⬟

2.5 ml/¹/₂ tsp salt

10 ml/2 tsp xanthum gum

10 ml/2 tsp gluten-free baking powder

30 ml/2 tbsp sunflower or olive oil

175 ml/6 fl oz/³/₄ cup dairy-free milk 🥄

60 ml/4 tbsp tomato purée (paste) or Red Lentil Sauce (see page 175)

100 g/4 oz/1 cup grated No-allergen Hard Cheese (see page 178) 🥄

2.5 ml/¹/₂ tsp dried oregano

2 × 105 g/4¹/₄ oz/small cans of skippers (brisling) in oil, drained

A mixed salad and Cool Coleslaw (see page 172), to serve

1 Mix the flour, salt, gum and baking powder together. Add the oil and milk and mix to form a soft but not sticky dough. Knead gently on a surface dusted with a little more wheat-free/gluten-free flour.

2 Divide the dough into four pieces. Roll out to four rounds, about 18 cm/6 in across. Transfer to an oiled baking (cookie) sheet.

3 Spread with the tomato purée or lentil sauce, then sprinkle with the cheese and oregano. Finally, arrange the skippers in a starburst pattern over the surfaces.

4 Bake in a preheated oven at 200°C/400°F/gas mark 6 (fan oven 180°C) for about 15 minutes until the edges are crisp and golden and the topping is bubbling. Serve hot.

Tolerant to ...	Variations
↖ Wheat	Use plain (all-purpose) flour instead of the wheat-free/gluten-free mix and omit the gum.
🥛 Dairy	Use cows' milk – full-cream for under-5s, semi-skimmed for older children – and Cheddar or ordinary Mozzarella.

Falafels

These are also delicious cold for a packed lunch with sticks of carrot or cucumber or cherry tomatoes.

MAKES 20

---

1 large onion, quartered

425 g/15 oz/1 large can of chick peas (garbanzos), drained

1 garlic clove, crushed

5 ml/1 tsp ground coriander (cilantro)

5 ml/1 tsp ground cumin

15 ml/1 tbsp chopped fresh parsley

15 ml/1 tbsp potato flour

40 g/1½ oz/⅓ cup rice flour ❧

60 ml/4 tbsp dairy-free milk 🌱 ☁

Oil, for deep-frying

Fresh Tomato or Cucumber Salsa (see page 170) and salad stuffs of your choice, to serve

1 Roughly chop the onion in a food processor.

2 Add the chick peas and garlic and run the machine until fairly smooth, stopping and scraping down the sides as necessary.

3 Stir in the spices, herbs and potato flour.

4 Shape into 20 small balls. Roll in the rice flour, then the milk, then the rice flour again. Chill for at least 30 minutes.

5 Deep-fry the balls in hot oil for about 3 minutes, turning once until crisp and golden. Drain on kitchen paper (paper towels). Serve warm with Fresh Tomato or Cucumber Salsa and salad.

Tolerant to ...	Variations
Eggs	Use 1 beaten egg instead of the milk, if liked.
Dairy	Use cows' milk – full-cream for under-5s, semi-skimmed for older children.
Wheat	Use plain (all-purpose) instead of rice flour.

Kids' Kedgeree

SERVES 4

225 g/8 oz/1 cup long-grain rice

1 large carrot, cut into small dice

225 g/8 oz smoked or white fish fillet, such as haddock

50 g/2 oz/¹/₂ cup frozen peas

15 g/¹/₂ oz/1 tbsp dairy-free margarine

Salt and freshly ground black pepper

15 ml/1 tbsp chopped fresh parsley (optional)

1 Cook the rice and carrot in boiling water for 3 minutes. Add the fish and peas and cook for a further 8 minutes or until the fish and rice are tender.

2 Lift out the fish. Drain the rice and peas and return them to the pan.

3 Remove the skin from the fish, break the flesh into small pieces, discarding any bones.

4 Stir the margarine into the rice until melted, then gently stir in the fish. Season lightly.

5 Spoon the mixture into warm bowls. Sprinkle with the parsley, if using, and serve hot.

Tolerant to ...	Variations
Dairy	Use butter or ordinary margarine.

Hot Potato and Bean Sauté

If your child is allergic to sweetcorn (corn), use peas or red kidney beans instead. If he can't have soy sauce, use gluten-free Worcestershire sauce or half the quantity of balsamic vinegar and a sprinkling of salt.

SERVES 4

---

700 g/1½ lb new potatoes, scraped or scrubbed and cut into even-sized pieces

Salt

50 g/2 oz/¼ cup dairy-free margarine 🌱

30 ml/2 tbsp sunflower oil

1 bunch of spring onions (scallions), cut into short lengths

1 green (bell) pepper, cut into thin strips

1 red pepper, cut into thin strips

350 g/12 oz/1 large can of sweetcorn (corn), drained

2.5 ml/½ tsp dried oregano

10 ml/2 tsp paprika

30 ml/2 tbsp gluten-free soy sauce

30 ml/2 tbsp chopped fresh parsley (optional)

Gluten-free tomato ketchup (catsup) or Brown Table Sauce (see page 166), to serve

1 Boil the potatoes in lightly salted water for about 8–10 minutes until just tender. Drain.

2 Melt the margarine and the oil in a large frying pan (skillet). Add the spring onions and peppers and fry (sauté), stirring, for 2 minutes. Add the potatoes and cook, tossing lightly for about 5 minutes until turning golden.

3 Add the sweetcorn, oregano, paprika and soy sauce and continue to cook, tossing gently for 5 minutes.

4 Pile on warm plates, sprinkle with parsley, if liked, and serve with ketchup or Brown Table Sauce.

Tolerant to ...	Variations
Dairy	Use butter or ordinary margarine.

Popeye's Ravioli

If your child can't have tomatoes, use the Red Lentil Sauce on page 175. Use guar gum instead of xanthum gum if corn cannot be tolerated.

SERVES 4

For the pasta:

175 g/6 oz/1½ cups Wheat-free/Gluten-free Flour Mix (see page 164) ✎

7.5 ml/1½ tsp xanthum gum

2.5 ml/½ tsp salt

15 ml/1 tbsp No Egg egg replacer (see page 20) ○

90 ml/6 tbsp warm water

15 ml/1 tbsp sunflower oil

A little rice flour, for dusting ✎

For the filling:

225 g/8 oz/1 small can of red kidney beans, drained

100 g/4 oz frozen chopped spinach, thawed

2.5 ml/½ tsp Marmite or other yeast extract

Freshly ground black pepper

For the sauce:

200 ml/7 fl oz/scant 1 cup passata (sieved tomatoes)

10 ml/2 tsp arrowroot

100 ml/3½ fl oz/scant ½ cup dairy-free milk ✦

10 ml/2 tsp tomato purée (paste)

2.5 ml/½ tsp caster (superfine) sugar

1.5 ml/¼ tsp dried basil

1 Mix the flour with the gum and salt in a bowl. Beat the egg replacer with the water until frothy. Add to the flour with the oil and mix to form a firm dough, adding a little extra water, if necessary.

2 Knead gently on a surface dusted with rice flour. Wrap the dough in clingfilm (plastic wrap) and leave to rest for 30 minutes.

3 Chop all the ingredients for the filling in a food processor. (Alternatively, put the drained beans in a bowl and mash thoroughly with a fork. Squeeze the spinach to remove excess water and add to the beans. Work together with the Marmite and pepper until well blended.)

4 Cut the dough in half and roll out each piece to a thin rectangle, about 20 × 25 cm/8 × 10 in. Put teaspoonfuls of the spinach mixture at 2 cm/^{3}/$_4$ in intervals across one piece of dough. Brush round each pile of filling with water.

5 Lay the second sheet of dough on top and press gently between each mound to seal. Cut between the mounds, using a sharp knife or pastry wheel.

6 Bring a large pan of lightly salted water to the boil. Drop in the ravioli and cook for 8 minutes until tender.

7 Meanwhile, put the passata in a saucepan. Blend the arrowroot with the milk and stir in. Add the tomato purée, sugar and basil and season lightly. Bring to the boil, stirring until slightly thickened.

8 Remove the ravioli from the pan with a draining spoon and transfer to bowls. Spoon the sauce over and serve.

Tolerant to ...	Variations
✎ Wheat	Use plain (all-purpose) flour instead of the wheat-free/gluten-free flour mix and the rice flour and omit the xanthum gum.
☺ Eggs	Use 2 large eggs, beaten, instead of the egg replacer and omit the water.
🥛 Dairy	Use cows' milk – full-cream for under-5s, semi-skimmed for older children.

DESSERTS

I'd encourage eating fresh fruit for pudding most of the time, but there are times when the dessert course needs to be a bit more special. And when you can't rely on a pot of mousse or even an ordinary yoghurt, life can be a bit tricky! Fruit desserts and rice, tapioca and sago puddings can easily be made with dairy-free milk, but pies, custards, mousses and many more favourites may cause problems. This chapter gives you tartlets and crumbles, trifles and even a fruity fromage frais for your child to enjoy.

JELLY, CUSTARD AND CREAM

Jelly (jello) tablets are a great standby for many desserts. If you are worried about the sugar content, you can buy sugar-free crystals although these do have artificial sweeteners in them. For the most part, I tend to use natural juice and gelatine to make jellies – 15 g/½ oz/ 1 tbsp of gelatine will set 600 ml/1 pt/2½ cups of pure fruit juice.

Beware of custard: it often has wheat flour in it as well as cornflour so buy gluten-free custard powder if necessary. If your child can't tolerate corn, you can make custard with rice flour instead (see the recipe on page 184).

Ordinary cream, too, is out for children on dairy-free diets. You'll find some clever alternatives on pages 181–3, to accompany these delicious desserts.

Crunchy Apple and Orange Crumble

You can substitute 100 g/4 oz blackberries or raspberries for the oranges if your child can't eat citrus fruit.

SERVES 4
450 g/1 lb cooking (tart) apples
3 oranges
30 ml/2 tbsp water
50 g/2 oz/¼ cup caster (superfine) sugar
50 g/2 oz/½ cup rice flour ⬠
25 g/1 oz/2 tbsp dairy-free margarine 🥄
50 g/2 oz/½ cup buckwheat grains ⬠
50 g/2 oz/¼ cup soft light brown sugar

1 Peel, quarter, core and slice the apples and place in an ovenproof dish. Hold the oranges, one at a time, over the apples in the dish. Cut off all the pith and cut into segments. Add the segments to the apples. Squeeze the membranes over to extract any remaining juice, then discard. Sprinkle with the caster sugar.

2 Put the rice flour in a bowl. Add the margarine and rub in with your fingertips. Stir in the buckwheat grains and the brown sugar. Sprinkle over the fruit and press down lightly.

3 Place on a baking (cookie) sheet and bake in a preheated oven at 190°C/375°F/gas mark 5 (fan oven 170°C) for about 45 minutes until golden and the apples are tender. Serve warm.

Tolerant to ...	Variations
⬠ Wheat	Use 100 g/4 oz/1 cup plain (all-purpose) flour instead of the combined rice flour and buckwheat grains.
🥄 Dairy	Use butter or ordinary margarine.

Mince Pies

It's best to make the mincemeat at least a week before you want to use it, to allow the flavours to develop. Place it in a sealed clean container and store in a cool, dry place.

MAKES ABOUT 24

---

100 g/4 oz/1 cup gluten-free shredded (chopped) vegetable suet

1 eating (dessert) apple, grated

450 g/1 lb dried mixed fruit (fruit cake mix)

100 g/4 oz/½ cup demerara sugar

100 g/4 oz/1 cup glacé (candied) cherries, quartered ☺

Finely grated zest and juice of 1 lemon

60 ml/4 tbsp orange juice

2.5 ml/½ tsp ground cinnamon

2.5 ml/½ tsp grated nutmeg

2.5 ml/½ tsp ground mace

1.5 ml/¼ tsp ground cloves

1 quantity of Dairy-free/Gluten-free Sweet Pastry (see page 165) ✎

Rice flour, for dusting ✎

Oil, for greasing

Dairy-free milk or water and caster (superfine) sugar, for glazing ✎

---

1   Mix the suet, apple, dried fruit, sugar, cherries, lemon zest and juice, orange juice and spices together, cover and leave to stand for at least 4 hours – preferably longer (see above).

2 Cut the pastry (paste) in half. Roll out on a surface dusted with rice flour and cut into rounds, using a 7.5 cm/3 in biscuit (cookie) cutter. Re-knead and roll the trimmings and use a little of the remaining pastry, if necessary, to make 24 rounds.

3 Roll out the remainder and cut slightly smaller rounds for 'lids'.

4 Press the larger rounds into the lightly greased sections of two tartlet tins (patty pans). Fill with mincemeat and top with pastry lids. Brush with milk or water and sprinkle with caster sugar.

5 Bake in a preheated oven at 200°C/400°F/gas mark 6 (fan oven 180°C) for about 20 minutes until golden brown. Cool slightly, then remove from the tin and cool on a wire rack.

Tolerant to ...	Variations
Nuts	Substitute half or all the glacé cherries with chopped mixed nuts, if liked.
Wheat	Use your usual shortcrust pastry (basic pie crust) recipe, made with half white vegetable fat and half dairy-free margarine, if necessary. Use plain (all-purpose) flour for dusting.
Dairy	Use cows' milk – full-cream for under-5s, semi-skimmed for older children.

Cherry Bakewell Tart

*If your child is allergic to citrus fruit, use an extra 15 ml/
1 tbsp water for the icing and omit the lemon juice.*

SERVES 6

---

*½ quantity of Dairy-free/Gluten-free Sweet Pastry
(see page 165)* ⬥ 🎗

....

45–60 ml/3–4 tbsp raspberry jam (conserve)

....

*½ quantity of Vanilla Sponge Cake mixture
(see page 130)* ⬥ 🎗 ◯ 🍪

....

175 g/6 oz/1 cup icing (confectioners') sugar

....

15 ml/1 tbsp lemon juice

....

15 ml/1 tbsp water

Glacé (candied) cherries, halved, for decorating

....

1 Roll out the pastry (paste) and use to line a 20 cm/8 in
   flan dish (pie pan), then place on a baking (cookie)
   sheet. Spread the base with the jam.

2 Make up the cake mixture, but substitute almond
   essence for the vanilla.

3 Spread over the jam and bake in a preheated oven at
   180°C/350°F/gas mark 4 (fan oven 160°C) for 25–30
   minutes until pale golden brown, cooked through and
   firm to the touch.

4 Leave to cool, then mix the icing sugar with the lemon
   juice and water to a thick, creamy consistency. Spread
   over the sponge and decorate with glacé cherries. Leave
   to set.

Tolerant to ...	Variations
Wheat	Use your own sweet shortcrust pastry (basic pie crust) recipe, made with dairy-free margarine and white vegetable fat, if necessary. Use self-raising (self-rising) flour instead of the speciality flours in the sponge.
Dairy	Use butter or ordinary margarine in the pastry and the cake mix.
Eggs	Use eggs in the sponge (see page 130).
Nuts	Use almond essence instead of vanilla.

Jam Tarts

MAKES 12

⅓ quantity of Dairy-free/Gluten-free Sweet Pastry (see page 165)

Rice flour, for dusting

Jam (conserve) of your choice

1 Roll out the pastry (paste) on a surface dusted with rice flour and cut into 12 rounds using a 7.5 cm/3 in biscuit (cookie) cutter. Press into the lightly greased sections of a tartlet tin (patty pan).

2 Add a good 5 ml/1 tsp of jam to each tart.

3 Bake in a preheated oven at 190°C/375°F/gas mark 5 (fan oven 170°C) for 15–20 minutes until golden brown. Cool slightly, then transfer to a wire rack to cool completely.

Tolerant to ...	Variations
Wheat	Use your ordinary shortcrust pastry (basic pie crust) recipe, made with half white vegetable fat and half dairy-free margarine, if necessary, and use plain (all-purpose) flour for dusting.

Chocolate or Carob Pudding with Sauce

If your child can't eat corn, use rice flour for the chocolate sauce and guar gum instead of xanthum gum. If he can't have lemon juice, use 10 ml/2 tsp of water and 5 ml/1 tsp of white wine vinegar instead.

SERVES 6

---

250 g/9 oz/generous 1 cup caster (superfine) sugar

175 g/6 oz/1½ cups wheat-free/gluten-free flour mix ↖

40 g/1½ oz/⅓ cup pure carob or cocoa (unsweetened chocolate) powder

7.5 ml/1½ tsp xanthum gum

5 ml/1 tsp bicarbonate of soda (baking soda)

2.5 ml/½ tsp instant coffee granules

15 ml/1 tbsp lemon juice

75 ml/5 tbsp sunflower oil

7.5 ml/1½ tsp natural vanilla essence (extract)

500 ml/17 fl oz/2¼ cups dairy-free milk ❦

30 ml/2 tbsp cornflour (cornstarch)

A little icing (confectioners') sugar, for dusting

---

1 Put 225 g/8 oz/1 cup of the sugar in a bowl. Sift in the flour, 25 g/1 oz/¼ cup of the carob or cocoa powder, the gum and bicarbonate of soda and stir into the sugar.

2 Dissolve the coffee in the lemon juice and add to the bowl with the oil, 5 ml/1 tsp of the vanilla essence and 250 ml/8 fl oz/1 cup of the milk. Beat until smooth.

3 Turn the mixture into an ungreased 1.2 litre/2 pt/5 cup ovenproof serving dish. Bake in a preheated oven at 180°C/350°F/gas mark 4 (fan oven 160°C) for about 35 minutes until the centre springs back when lightly pressed.

4 Meanwhile, blend the cornflour with the remaining carob or cocoa powder in a small saucepan. Add the remaining sugar, then blend in the remaining milk. Bring to the boil and cook for 1 minute, stirring until thickened and smooth. Add the remaining vanilla essence.

5 Dust the pudding with icing sugar and serve hot with the sauce.

Tolerant to ...	Variations
🍷 Dairy	Use cows' milk – full-cream for under-5s, semi-skimmed for older children.
↘ Wheat	Use plain (all-purpose) flour instead of the flour mix and omit the xanthum gum.

Banana and Caramel Velvet

SERVES 4

100 g/4 oz/¹/₂ cup granulated sugar

30 ml/2 tbsp water

50 g/2 oz/¹/₄ cup dairy-free margarine 🥛

30 ml/2 tbsp arrowroot

600 ml/1 pt/2¹/₂ cups dairy-free milk 🥛

4 small or 2 large bananas, sliced

5 ml/1 tsp lemon juice (optional)

Coloured sugar strands, for decorating

1 Put the sugar and water in a heavy-based saucepan. Heat gently, stirring, until the sugar dissolves. Bring to the boil and boil rapidly until the mixture is a golden brown.

2 Remove from the heat and leave to cool slightly. Stir in the margarine.

3 Blend the arrowroot with a little of the milk in a small bowl. Stir the remaining milk into the sugar mixture and stir over a gentle heat until blended and all the caramel has melted.

4 Blend in the arrowroot mixture and bring to the boil, stirring until thickened. Remove from the heat. Cover with a circle of wet greaseproof (waxed) paper and leave to cool.

5 Toss the banana slices in lemon juice to prevent browning, if liked. Divide among four sundae glasses. Spoon the cold caramel custard over and chill. Sprinkle with coloured sugar strands just before serving.

Tolerant to ...	Variations
♥ Dairy	Use cows' milk – full-cream for under-5s, semi-skimmed for older children – and ordinary butter or margarine.

Jelly Cloud

Serve this with matching canned or fresh fruit, if liked.

SERVES 4
---

1 tablet of any fruit-flavoured jelly (jello)

Boiling water

Ice cubes or cold water

300 ml/½ pt/1¼ cups dairy-free milk ♥

1 Break up the jelly tablet and place it in a measuring jug. Top up to 200 ml/7 fl oz/scant 1 cup with boiling water and stir until dissolved.

2 Add ice cubes or cold water to the jelly, to make it up to 300 ml/½ pt/1¼ cups. Leave until cool but not setting.

3 Stir in the cold milk. Pour into a wetted jelly mould or individual glasses and chill until set.

Tolerant to ...	Variations
♥ Dairy	Use cows' milk – full-cream for under-5s, semi-skimmed for older children.

Syrup Tartlets

You can use the same quantities to make 1 large (20 cm/8 in) tart, on a pie plate, if you prefer. In the US, if your child can't tolerate corn, use maple syrup or clear honey instead of light corn syrup.

MAKES 12

½ quantity of Dairy-free/Gluten-free Sweet Pastry (see page 165) ⬞

Rice flour, for dusting ⬞

60 ml/4 tbsp wheat- and gluten-free breadcrumbs (use any of the breads on pages 117–24) ⬞

A good 60 ml/4 tbsp golden (light corn) syrup

Finely grated zest of ½ lemon (optional)

1 Roll out the pastry (paste) on a surface dusted with rice flour and cut into 12 rounds using a 7.5 cm/3 in biscuit (cookie) cutter.

2 Press into the greased sections of a tartlet tin (patty pan).

3 Spoon the breadcrumbs into each case and top each with a good 5 ml/1 tsp of syrup, then scatter over the lemon zest, if using.

4 Bake in a preheated oven at 190°C/375°F/gas mark 5 (fan oven 170°C) for about 20 minutes until golden and bubbling. Remove from the tin and serve warm or cold.

Tolerant to ...	Variations
⬞ Wheat	Use your ordinary shortcrust pastry (basic pie crust) recipe, using half white vegetable fat and half dairy-free margarine, if necessary. Use ordinary breadcrumbs. Dust the surface with plain (all-purpose) flour.

Traffic Lights

The selection of green, orange and red fruits is up to you (and your child's preferences). For the green fruit, you could use greengages, halved and stoned, or green grapes, or an avocado, cut into chunks. For orange, you could use a segmented orange or a persimmon, cut into chunks, and for red, large strawberries or stoned red cherries, or a red apple, cut into chunks. If your child can't eat any yoghurts, make this Raspberry Dip: purée a drained can of raspberries in natural juice, then rub the purée through a sieve to remove the seeds. Sweeten and thicken slightly with a little sifted icing sugar.

SERVES 4

1 kiwi fruit, cut into 8 chunks

1 small mango, cut into 8 chunks

1 wedge of water melon, cut into 8 chunks

For the dip:

250 ml/8 fl oz/1 cup plain sheep's yoghurt 🌡 ᠙

30 ml/2 tbsp clear honey

A pinch of ground cinnamon (optional)

---

1 Thread a piece of green fruit on each of eight cocktail sticks (toothpicks), then add a piece of orange fruit, then a piece of red fruit.

2 Mix the yoghurt with the honey and cinnamon, if using, and spoon into small pots. Serve the kebabs with the dip.

Tolerant to ...	Variations
🌡 Dairy	Use cows' milk yoghurt.
᠙ Soya	Use soya yoghurt.

Pineapple Trifle

This is a great way of using up a little stale left-over Vanilla Sponge Cake (see page 130) or any allergen-free plain biscuits. If your child is allergic to corn, use rice flour in the Cornmeal Custard on page 184.

SERVES 4

100 g/4 oz stale Vanilla Sponge Cake or any plain dairy-free/gluten-free biscuits (cookies) ☻ ✎

60 ml/4 tbsp red jam (conserve), any flavour

225 g/8 oz/1 small can of pineapple pieces, drained, reserving the juice

10 ml/2 tsp powdered gelatine

150 ml/¼ pt/⅔ cup pure apple juice

60 ml/4 tbsp gluten-free custard powder ✎

600 ml/1 pt/2½ cups dairy-free milk ☙

30 ml/2 tbsp caster (superfine) sugar

2 glacé (candied) cherries, halved

1 Crumble the cake or biscuits and divide among four sundae glasses.

2 Add a spoonful of jam to each glass.

3 Spoon the pineapple pieces over.

4 Put the gelatine and the pineapple juice in a small bowl. Leave to soften for 5 minutes, then dissolve either by placing the bowl in a pan of simmering water or by heating briefly in the microwave. Stir in the apple juice, then spoon over the pineapple. Chill until set.

5 Meanwhile, blend the custard powder with a little of the milk and the sugar in a saucepan. Stir in the remaining milk. Bring to the boil and cook, stirring, for 1 minute until thickened.

6 Cover with a circle of wet greaseproof (waxed) paper and leave to cool. Spoon the custard over the jelly and chill until ready to serve, decorated with a half glacé cherry on top of each.

Tolerant to ...	Variations
🥛 Dairy	Use cows' milk – full-cream for under-5s, semi-skimmed for older children.
🌾 Wheat	Use ordinary cake or biscuits.
🥜 Nuts	Use macaroons instead of plain cake or biscuits.

Lime, Lemon or Orange Slush

If your child is allergic to citrus fruits, use a 225 g/
8 oz/small can of pineapple in natural juice, puréed in a
blender or food processor, instead.

SERVES 4–6

5 limes OR 4 lemons OR 4 oranges

15 ml/1 tbsp lemon juice (if using oranges)

300 ml/½ pt/1¼ cups water

175 g/6 oz/¾ cup caster (superfine) sugar

1 Squeeze all the juice from the fruit. Strain to remove any pips. If using oranges, stir in the lemon juice.

2 Add the water, then the sugar, stirring until completely dissolved.

3 Pour into a freezer-proof container and freeze for 2 hours. Whisk well with a fork and freeze for a further 2 hours. Whisk again and freeze until firm.

4 When ready to serve, break up roughly and tip into a blender or food processor. Run the machine until the mixture is slushy. Serve straight away.

Apricot Crisp

If your child is allergic to corn, use rice crispies instead of the cornflakes and in the US, use clear honey or maple syrup, not light corn syrup.

SERVES 4

---

425 g/15 oz/1 large can of apricots in natural juice

1 orange jelly (jello) tablet

300 ml/¹/₂ pt/1¹/₄ cups boiling water

150 ml/¹/₄ pt/²/₃ cup Whipped Rice Cream (see page 181) or plain dairy-free yoghurt ⬙

25 g/1 oz/2 tbsp dairy-free margarine ⬙

30 ml/2 tbsp golden (light corn) syrup

50 g/2 oz/1 cup cornflakes, lightly crushed

1 Purée the apricots and their juice in a blender or food processor.

2 Dissolve the jelly in the boiling water and stir into the fruit purée. Turn into four individual glass bowls and leave to set.

3 Spread the set fruit with the 'whipped cream' or yoghurt.

4 Melt the margarine with the syrup in a saucepan. Stir in the cornflakes. Leave to cool slightly, then spoon over the desserts and leave to cool. Chill until ready to serve.

Tolerant to ...	Variations
⬙ Dairy	Use butter or ordinary hard margarine and cows' milk cream or yoghurt.

Fruit Fromage Frais

Weigh the fruit after preparation. You can use bought soya, sheep's or goats' soft cheese, if your child can eat them.

SERVES 4

---

225 g/8 oz fresh ripe pears, raspberries, strawberries, peaches or nectarines, cored or stoned (pitted) as necessary

1 quantity of Non-dairy Soft Cheese (see page 180) 🥛

A little icing (confectioners') sugar

1 Purée the fruit in a blender or food processor. If liked, rub through a sieve (strainer) to remove any pips or skin.

2 Mix with the cheese until well blended, then sweeten to taste with icing sugar. Spoon into small pots and chill until ready to serve.

Tolerant to ...	Variations
🥛 Dairy	Use plain cows' milk fromage frais.

BREADS, BISCUITS AND CAKES

This is probably the most important chapter of all. Just about every kind of bread, biscuit (cookie) or cake you buy has potential allergens in it – mostly wheat/gluten, eggs and dairy products. You can, of course, make your own but even that's not entirely straightforward because, for example, you can't just substitute another flour with the same results because it's the gluten in wheat that creates the texture and distinctive flavour. You can buy a whole range of gluten-free bakes but they tend to be dull, disappointing and very expensive.

Gluten-free flour mix doesn't work well in yeast cookery (it's just not like real bread!) but you can now buy xanthum, sometimes called xanthan gum, which can be added to wheat-free/gluten-free flour mixes to give that delicious elasticity. It's good in other bakes, too, so even though it's expensive, it is worth buying (and a little goes a long way). It is made from corn, which means it can't be tolerated by some, but you can use guar gum in the same way although this isn't so readily available or so good.

However, you don't have to have gum for all the recipes. I've managed to create some excellent breads without it. I discovered that pectin has a similar effect to the gum and, after a lot of trial and error, I succeeded in creating a loaf using grated apple (high in pectin) to add the extra stretchy quality! I've also made another super yeast bread using rice flour and a delicious buckwheat soda bread.

Please note, however, if your child can tolerate wheat/gluten, there is little point in going to the effort of making special breads – commercially produced bread is unlikely to contain any real eggs or milk (apart from milk loaf, obviously).

As children, in particular, can't be expected not to want to eat biscuits and cakes, I've also developed a whole range of sweet treats for them to enjoy – and I do mean 'enjoy', not just put up with!

Crusty White Bread

You must grate the skin of the apple as well as the flesh, because the pectin, which helps the bread to rise, is just under it. I haven't added a variations box because, if you are not on a wheat-free/gluten-free diet, you can use any ordinary bread recipe, if necessary substituting sunflower oil or dairy-free margarine for any butter or margarine.

MAKES 1 SMALL LOAF

A little oil, for greasing

225 g/8 oz/2 cups wheat-free/gluten-free flour mix, plus a little for dusting

1 sachet of easy-blend dried yeast

2.5 ml/½ tsp salt

1 eating (dessert) apple

15 ml/1 tbsp sunflower oil

200 ml/7 fl oz/scant 1 cup hand-hot water

1 Grease a 450 g/1 lb loaf tin (pan) and dust with a little of the flour.

2 Put all the ingredients except the water in a large mixing bowl and mix well. Add the water and beat until the mixture forms a thick batter.

3 Turn into the prepared tin. Place in a warm place for 15 minutes until the dough almost reaches the top of the tin.

4 Stand the tin in a roasting tin containing about 2.5 cm/1 in of boiling water. Bake towards the top of a preheated oven at 200°C/400°F/gas mark 6 (fan oven 180°C) for 1 hour.

5 Turn out of the tin, place upside-down on the oven shelf and bake for a further 15 minutes to crisp the crust. Cool on a wire rack.

Large White Loaf

If your child is allergic to corn, remember to use guar gum, instead of xanthum gum. Use white wine vinegar instead of lemon juice if he can tolerate citrus fruit.

MAKES 1 LARGE LOAF

A little oil, for greasing

350 g/12 oz/3 cups wheat-free/gluten-free flour mix, plus extra for dusting

15 ml/1 tbsp xanthum gum

5 ml/1 tsp salt

1 sachet of easy-blend dried yeast

10 ml/2 tsp No Egg egg replacer (see page 20) ⌣

60 ml/4 tbsp warm water

75 ml/5 tbsp sunflower oil

150 ml/¹/₄ pt/²/₃ cup hand-hot dairy-free milk, plus a little for brushing 🥛

5 ml/1 tsp lemon juice

150 ml/¹/₄ pt/²/₃ cup hand-hot water

---

1 Grease a 900 g/2 lb loaf tin (pan) and dust with a little of the flour mix.

2 Sift the flour, gum and salt into a bowl or a food processor. Add the yeast.

3 Whisk the egg replacer and the measured warm water together until frothy.

4 Add to the flour mixture with the oil, milk, lemon juice and hand-hot water and beat with an electric or hand whisk or run the food processor for 2 minutes.

5 Spoon the mixture into the prepared tin and level the surface. Place in a warm place and leave to rise to the top of the tin. Brush the top very lightly with milk.

6 Bake in a preheated oven at 200°C/400°F/gas mark 6 (fan oven 180°C) for 40 minutes until risen and golden. Turn out of the tin and place upside-down on the oven shelf. Continue to cook for 10 minutes.

7 Transfer to a wire rack and leave to cool.

Tolerant to ...	Variations
⌒ Eggs	Substitute 2 eggs for the egg replacer and omit the 60 ml/4 tbsp of warm water.
❦ Dairy	Use cows' milk – full-cream for under-5s, semi-skimmed for older children.

Dairy-free Milk Loaf

*This loaf sometimes goes flat on the top when baked –
especially if it is slightly over-proved. However, it does not
spoil the texture so don't worry!*

MAKES 1 SMALL LOAF

A little oil, for greasing

5 ml/1 tsp No Egg egg replacer (see page 20) ⟁

30 ml/2 tbsp warm water

175 g/6 oz/1½ cups rice flour, plus a little for dusting

2.5 ml/½ tsp salt

10 ml/2 tsp caster (superfine) sugar

1 sachet of easy-blend dried yeast

15 ml/1 tbsp sunflower oil

150 ml/¼ pt/⅔ cup hand-hot dairy-free milk ▉

---

1 Grease a 450 g/1 lb loaf tin (pan) and dust with a little rice flour.

2 Whisk the egg replacer and warm water together until frothy.

3 Mix the rice flour, salt, sugar and yeast in a large bowl. Add the egg replacer, oil and milk and beat to form a thick batter.

4 Turn into the prepared tin and leave in a warm place for 20 minutes until the mixture almost reaches the top of the tin.

5 Place in a roasting tin containing 2.5 cm/1 in of boiling water. Bake in a preheated oven on a shelf just above the centre at 200°C/400°F/gas mark 6 (fan oven 180°C) for 20 minutes. Turn out of the tin, place upside-down on the oven shelf and cook for 10 minutes to crisp the crust. Cool on a wire rack.

Tolerant to ...	Variations
⌒ Eggs	Substitute 1 egg for the egg replacer and omit the warm water.
🍶 Dairy	Use cows' milk – full-cream for under-5s, semi-skimmed for older children.

Garlic and Herb Bread Slices

Most children seem to love garlic bread and this is a delicious alternative to the traditional baguette for those who can't eat it – and makes a change for those who can! You can use any of the breads on pages 117–24.

SERVES 4

25 g/1 oz/2 tbsp dairy-free margarine 🍶

15 ml/1 tbsp sunflower or olive oil

1–2 large garlic cloves, crushed

15 ml/1 tbsp chopped fresh parsley

2.5 ml/½ tsp dried mixed herbs

Freshly ground black pepper

4 thick slices of wheat-free/gluten-free bread, cut in half diagonally ⟍

1 Heat the margarine and oil in a large frying pan (skillet). Add the garlic, herbs and some pepper.

2 Add the bread and turn over in the fat to coat completely. Cook over a gentle heat, turning once during cooking, until just beginning to brown round the edges on both sides but still fairly soft in the middle. Serve hot.

Tolerant to ...	Variations
⟍ Wheat	Use ordinary bread.
🍶 Dairy	Use butter or ordinary margarine.

Wheat-free/Gluten-free
Soft White Bread

For this recipe, I use the bought gluten-free white bread flour mix made by Dove Farms. Alternatively, make your own mix including tapioca flour (see page 164) and add 10 ml/2 tsp of xanthum gum to the flour mix (or guar gum if your child can't tolerate corn). I have added rice flour to this recipe as well, because I found that using just the bread mix made a very gluey loaf!

MAKES 1 SMALL LOAF

A little oil, for greasing

....

175 g/6 oz/1½ cups gluten-free white bread flour mix

....

50 g/2 oz/¼ cup rice flour, plus extra for dusting

....

4 ml/¾ tsp salt

....

4 ml/¾ tsp caster (superfine) sugar

....

10 ml/2 tsp easy-blend dried yeast

....

5 ml/1 tsp lemon juice

....

30 ml/2 tbsp sunflower oil

....

175 ml/6 fl oz/¾ cup dairy-free milk 🍃

....

60 ml/4 tbsp water

....

1 Grease a 450 g/1 lb loaf tin (pan) and dust with a little rice flour.

2 Sift the bread flour mix and rice flour together with the salt and sugar into a large bowl.

3 Add the yeast, lemon juice and sunflower oil.

4 Heat the milk and water together until hand-hot. Add to the bowl and beat well with an electric beater or balloon whisk until smooth.

5 Spoon into the prepared tin and level the surface. Leave in a warm place until the dough reaches the top of the tin.

6 Stand the tin in a roasting tin containing 2.5 cm/1 in of boiling water. Bake in a preheated oven at 180°C/ 350°F/gas mark 4 (fan oven 160°C) for 40 minutes. Leave in the tin for 15 minutes, then turn out on to a wire rack to cool, covered with a damp tea towel (dish cloth) to keep the crust soft.

Tolerant to ...	Variations
🥛 Dairy	Use cows' milk – full-cream for under-5s, semi-skimmed for older children.

Soda Bread

A little oil, for greasing

100 g/4 oz/1 cup buckwheat flour, plus a little for dusting ⬎

100 g/4 oz/1 cup rice flour ⬎

5 ml/1 tsp bicarbonate of soda (baking soda)

5 ml/1 tsp cream of tartar

5 ml/1 tsp caster (superfine) sugar

2.5 ml/½ tsp salt

15 g/½ oz/1 tbsp dairy-free margarine 🍯

300 ml/½ pt/1¼ cups dairy-free milk 🍯

1 Grease a 450 g/1 lb loaf tin (pan) or deep, round 15 cm/6 in cake tin. Dust with a little buckwheat flour.

2 Mix the flours with the bicarbonate of soda, cream of tartar, sugar and salt. Rub in the margarine.

3 Mix with the milk and beat well to form a thick batter.

4 Pour into the prepared tin. Bake in a preheated oven at 200°C/400°F/gas mark 6 (fan oven 180°C) for 30–40 minutes until the loaf is risen and browned and the base sounds hollow when tipped out and tapped.

Tolerant to ...	Variations
⬎ Wheat	Use 225 g/8 oz/2 cups plain (all-purpose) or wholemeal flour instead of the buckwheat and rice flour.
🍯 Dairy	Use butter or ordinary margarine and cows' milk – full-cream for under-5s, semi-skimmed for older children.

Savoury Crackers

These are nice on their own or topped with a savoury spread for a snack meal.

MAKES ABOUT 18

100 g/4 oz/1 cup buckwheat flour ↖

100 g/4 oz/1 cup rice flour, plus extra for dusting ↖

2.5 ml/¹/₂ tsp onion or celery salt

5 ml/1 tsp bicarbonate of soda (baking soda)

150 g/5 oz/²/₃ cup dairy-free margarine 🥛

A little water

1 Sift the flours, flavoured salt and bicarbonate of soda into a bowl. Work in the margarine with a fork.

2 Add water, if necessary, a drop at a time, to form a soft but not sticky dough.

3 Knead gently on a surface dusted with rice flour. Roll out thinly to a rectangle, then cut into 5 cm/2 in squares. Transfer to a lightly greased baking (cookie) sheet.

4 Bake in a preheated oven at 180°C/350°F/gas mark 4 (fan oven 160°C) for about 30 minutes until lightly browned. Leave to cool slightly, then transfer to a wire rack to cool completely. Store in an airtight container.

Tolerant to ...	Variations
↖ Wheat	Use half wholemeal and half plain (all-purpose) flour instead of the buckwheat and rice flours.
🥛 Dairy	Use butter or ordinary margarine.

Rusks

When your baby is teething and can hold things himself, rusks are a good food to gnaw on. They are also popular with older children, spread with a little margarine (dairy-free, if necessary) and Marmite, my Apple and Date Spread (see page 179) or other toppings of their choice. Make some when you are baking something else – it's a great way to use up a stale loaf.
Remember, never leave your baby alone when eating.

MAKES UP TO 24

---

4 large or 6 small thick slices of wheat-free/gluten-free bread ❧

75 ml/5 tbsp dairy-free milk or formula milk ♥

1 Cut each slice into three or four fingers.

2 Dip in the milk to coat both sides.

3 Place on a non-stick baking (cookie) sheet or an ordinary baking sheet covered with a piece of non-stick baking parchment.

4 Bake in a preheated oven at 180°C/350°F/gas mark 4 (fan oven 160°C) for about 45 minutes to 1 hour until crisp, dry and golden. Leave to cool, then store in an airtight container.

Tolerant to ...	Variations
♥ Dairy	Use full-cream cows' milk.
❧ Wheat	Use ordinary bread.

Tortillas

These are tasty at any time, even breakfast, spread with margarine (dairy-free, if necessary) and a little Marmite or honey. If your child can't tolerate corn, you can omit the maize and use all flour mix but the texture won't be so good.

MAKES 8

---

100 g/4 oz/1 cup wheat-free/gluten-free flour mix ✎

50 g/2 oz/½ cup maize meal

1.5 ml/¼ tsp salt

5 ml/1 tsp No Egg egg replacer (see page 20) ☾

30 ml/2 tbsp warm water

200 ml/7 fl oz/scant 1 cup cold water

A little sunflower oil, for greasing

1 Mix the flour, maize meal and salt together in a bowl.

2 Whisk the egg replacer and warm water together until frothy. Add to the bowl with the cold water and beat to form a smooth batter.

3 Lightly grease an omelette pan with oil, wiping out any excess. Heat the pan. Spoon in about 30 ml/2 tbsp of the batter and swirl quickly to coat the base of the pan. Cook over a moderate heat until slightly curling at the edges and drying out.

4 Turn and cook the other side briefly. Slide out on to a plate and keep warm, wrapped in kitchen paper (paper towels), while cooking the remainder.

Tolerant to ...	Variations
✎ Wheat	Use plain (all-purpose) flour.
☾ Eggs	Use 1 beaten egg instead of the egg replacer and omit the warm water.

Doughnut Trails

These taste very like churros – the Spanish-style doughnut strips. Remember to use guar gum instead of xanthum gum if your child is allergic to corn.

MAKES ABOUT 12

---

100 g/4 oz/1 cup rice flour ✎

5 ml/1 tsp xanthum gum

A pinch of salt

60 ml/4 tbsp caster (superfine) sugar

10 ml/2 tsp gluten-free baking powder

175 ml/6 fl oz/³/₄ cup dairy-free milk ☙

Oil, for deep-frying

2.5 ml/¹/₂ tsp ground cinnamon (optional)

---

1 Sift the flour, gum, salt, 10 ml/2 tsp of the sugar and the baking powder together. Whisk in the milk to form a paste.

2 Heat oil for deep-frying to 190°C/375°F or until a cube of day-old bread (remember to use gluten-free if necessary) browns in 30 seconds. Put the dough either in a piping bag with a large star tube (tip) or in a plastic bag with the corner of the bag snipped off. Pipe the dough into the hot oil, cutting it off at about 7.5 cm/3 in intervals.

3 Cook, turning over as necessary, for about 3 minutes or until golden brown and cooked through. Remove with a draining spoon and drain on kitchen paper (paper towels). Place the pieces in a bag with the remaining sugar and the cinnamon, if using. Hold the bag closed and shake it to coat the doughnuts. Serve whilst very fresh.

Tolerant to ...	Variations
↖ Wheat	Use plain (all-purpose) flour instead of the rice flour and omit the gum.
🥛 Dairy	Use cows' milk – full-cream for under-5s, semi-skimmed milk for older children.

Honeyed Cereal Bars

When I created the delicious cereal on page 47, it gave me the idea for a cereal bar along the same lines!

MAKES 12

50 g/2 oz/¼ cup dairy-free margarine 🥛

100 g/4 oz/1 small packet of marshmallows

30 ml/2 tbsp clear honey

100 g/4 oz/2 cups rice crispies

100 g/4 oz/1 cup buckwheat grains

100 g/2 oz/⅓ cup raisins

10 ml/2 tsp ground mixed (apple-pie) spice

A little oil, for greasing

1 Put the margarine, marshmallows and honey in a heavy-based saucepan and heat gently, stirring, until melted.

2 Stir in the cereals, raisins and spice.

3 Using the back of a wet spoon, press firmly into an oiled 18 × 28 cm/7 × 11 in shallow baking tin (pan).

4 Leave until cold and set firm, then cut into fingers. Store in an airtight container.

Tolerant to ...	Variations
🥛 Dairy	Use butter or ordinary hard margarine.

Vanilla Sponge Cake

You can use gram flour instead of rice flour for this recipe. It is very nutritious and gives a great texture, but it has a distinct taste of dried peas. You can disguise the flavour by adding 15 ml/1 tbsp of instant coffee powder or pure carob or cocoa powder, blended with 30 ml/2 tbsp of warm water.

MAKES ONE 18 CM/7 IN CAKE

A little oil, for greasing

35 ml/7 tsp No Egg egg replacer (see page 20) ⬭

120 ml/4 fl oz/¹/₂ cup warm water

150 g/5 oz/²/₃ cup soft light brown sugar

1.5 ml/¹/₄ tsp natural vanilla essence (extract)

75 g/3 oz/¹/₃ cup dairy-free margarine, melted 🍶

75 g/3 oz/³/₄ cup rice flour ⬎ 👄

75 g/3 oz/³/₄ cup potato flour ⬎

10 ml/2 tsp gluten-free baking powder

A little caster (superfine) sugar, for dusting

1 Grease a deep, round 18 cm/7 in cake tin (pan) and line with non-stick baking parchment or greased greaseproof (waxed) paper.

2 Whisk the egg replacer and water together in a large bowl with an electric or balloon whisk until white, glossy and softly peaking. Add the sugar and vanilla and whisk until the mixture is thick and the whisk leaves a trail when lifted out.

3 Gradually whisk the margarine into the mixture. Sift the flours and baking powder over and fold in.

4 Turn into the prepared tin. Bake in a preheated oven at 160°C/325°F/gas mark 3 (fan oven 145°C) for about 40 minutes until the cake is risen and golden and the centre springs back when lightly pressed.

5 Cool slightly, then turn out on to a wire rack, remove the paper and leave to cool.

6 Dust with caster sugar before serving.

Tolerant to ...	Variations
☞ Soya	Use soya flour instead of the rice flour.
✎ Wheat	Use plain (all-purpose) flour instead of the rice and potato flours.
☁ Eggs	Use 3 eggs instead of the egg replacer and omit the warm water. Lightly beat, then add the sugar and whisk until thick. Fold in the sifted flours, then, lastly, fold in the melted margarine.
♥ Dairy	Use butter or ordinary margarine.

Jam Sponge Cake

MAKES ONE 18 CM/7 IN CAKE

Prepare as for Vanilla Sponge Cake (above), with variations as necessary. When cold, split the cake in half horizontally and sandwich the layers together again with about 45 ml/3 tbsp of your favourite jam (conserve).

Vanilla Buttercream Sponge Cake

MAKES ONE 18 CM/7 IN CAKE

Prepare the Vanilla Sponge Cake (above), with variations as necessary. Make a 'buttercream' by beating 50 g/2 oz/¼ cup of margarine (dairy-free, if necessary) with a few drops of natural vanilla essence (extract) and 150 g/5 oz/scant 1 cup of sifted icing (confectioners') sugar until smooth. Use half to fill the cake and add jam (conserve), too, if liked. Spread the remainder on top and decorate with the prongs of a fork.

Carob or Chocolate Cupcakes

MAKES 12

100 g/4 oz/¹/₂ cup dairy-free margarine 🥄

100 g/4 oz/¹/₂ cup soft light brown sugar

10 ml/2 tsp No Egg egg replacer (see page 20) ⌒

120 ml/4 fl oz/¹/₂ cup warm water

125 g/4¹/₂ oz/generous 1 cup wheat-free/gluten-free flour mix ↖

10 ml/2 tsp gluten-free baking powder

50 g/2 oz/¹/₂ cup pure carob or cocoa (unsweetened chocolate) powder

225 g/8 oz/1¹/₃ cups icing (confectioners') sugar

1 Put the margarine and sugar in a bowl and beat until light and fluffy.

2 Beat the egg replacer with 60 ml/4 tbsp of the water until frothy. Add to the mixture and beat thoroughly.

3 Sift the flour, baking powder and half the carob or cocoa powder over the surface and fold in with a metal spoon. Stir in 30 ml/2 tbsp of the remaining water to form a very soft, dropping consistency.

4 Spoon into 12 paper cake cases (cupcake papers) in a tartlet tin (patty pan). Level the surfaces.

5 Bake in a preheated oven at 190°C/375°F/gas mark 5 (fan oven 170°C) for 15–20 minutes until the cakes are risen and the centres spring back when lightly pressed. Transfer to a wire rack to cool.

6 Sift the icing sugar with the remaining carob or cocoa powder. Mix with enough of the remaining water to form a thick cream. Spread over the tops of the cooled cakes and leave to set.

Tolerant to ...	Variations
↖ Wheat	Use plain (all-purpose) flour.
◔ Eggs	Use 2 eggs instead of the egg replacer and omit the water. Lightly beat together before adding to the margarine and sugar.
🥛 Dairy	Use softened butter or ordinary margarine.

Chocolate Cherry Cracklers

If your child is allergic to corn, use rice crispies.

MAKES 12

---

50 g/2 oz/¼ cup dairy-free margarine 🥛

45 ml/3 tbsp clear honey

50 g/2 oz/¼ cup caster (superfine) sugar

50 g/2 oz/¼ cup glacé (candied) cherries, chopped

25 g/1 oz/2 tbsp pure carob or cocoa (unsweetened chocolate) powder, plus extra for dusting

100 g/4 oz/2 cups cornflakes, crushed

1 Melt the margarine, honey and sugar in a saucepan, stirring. Bring to the boil and boil for 1 minute.

2 Remove from the heat and stir in the cherries, carob or cocoa powder and cornflakes.

3 Spoon the mixture into paper cake cases (cupcake papers) and chill until firm. Dust with carob or cocoa powder before serving.

Tolerant to ...	Variations
🥛 Dairy	Use butter or ordinary margarine.

Moist Fruit Cake

A little oil, for greasing

175 g/6 oz/³/₄ cup dairy-free margarine, softened 🍶

175 g/6 oz/³/₄ cup soft light brown sugar

20 ml/4 tsp No Egg egg replacer (see page 20) 🥚

120 ml/4 fl oz/¹/₂ cup warm water

1 eating (dessert) apple, grated, including the skin

50 g/2 oz/¹/₂ cup gram flour ✎

50 g/2 oz/¹/₂ cup potato flour

100 g/4 oz/1 cup rice flour ✎

15 ml/1 tbsp gluten-free baking powder

5 ml/1 tsp ground cinnamon

5 ml/1 tsp mixed (apple-pie) spice

225 g/8 oz/1¹/₃ cups dried mixed fruit (fruit cake mix)

1 Grease and line a deep, round, loose-bottomed 18 cm/ 7 in cake tin (pan) with non-stick baking parchment or greased greaseproof (waxed) paper.

2 Beat the margarine and sugar together until light and fluffy.

3 Beat the egg replacer and water together until frothy. Beat into the margarine and sugar mixture, a little at a time. The mixture will curdle.

4 Beat in the apple, then sift the flours, baking powder and spices over the surface and fold in.

5 Add the fruit and fold in.

6 Turn into the prepared tin and level the surface. Bake in a preheated oven at 160°C/325°F/gas mark 3 (fan oven 145°C) for 1¼–1½ hours until it is a rich brown and a skewer inserted in the centre comes out clean. (Check after an hour and if it is over-browning, cover with foil.)

7 Leave to cool in the tin for 10 minutes, then turn out on to a wire rack, remove the paper and leave to cool completely.

Tolerant to ...	Variations
Wheat	Use plain (all-purpose) or wholemeal flour instead of the rice and gram flours.
Soya	Use soya flour instead of the gram flour.
Eggs	Use 3 large eggs instead of the egg replacer and omit the water. Lightly beat together, then add to the margarine mixture as in the recipe.
Dairy	Use softened butter or ordinary tub margarine.

Carob or Chocolate Slab Cake

MAKES 9 SQUARES

100 g/4 oz/1 cup wheat-free/gluten-free flour mix ↘

45 ml/3 tbsp pure carob or cocoa (unsweetened chocolate) powder

10 ml/2 tsp gluten-free baking powder

1.5 ml/¼ tsp salt

100 g/4 oz/½ cup granulated sugar

100 g/4 oz/½ cup dairy-free margarine ❦

105 ml/7 tbsp warm water

15 ml/1 tbsp No Egg egg replacer (see page 20) ○

5 ml/1 tsp natural vanilla essence (extract)

50 g/2 oz/½ cup dairy-free/gluten-free carob or plain (semi-sweet) chocolate, broken up

1 Grease a square, shallow 18 cm/7 in baking tin (pan) and line with non-stick baking parchment.

2 Sift the flour, carob or cocoa powder, baking powder and salt into a bowl.

3 Put the sugar, margarine and 30 ml/2 tbsp of the water in a saucepan and heat until melted.

4 Whisk the egg replacer with the remaining water until frothy. Add to the flour mixture with the melted mixture and the vanilla essence and beat well to form a smooth batter.

5 Pour into the prepared tin. Bake in a preheated oven at 190°C/375°F/gas mark 5 (fan oven 170°C) for 15–20 minutes until firm to the touch. Take care not to overcook or the cake will become too dry.

6 Leave to cool slightly, then transfer to a wire rack to cool completely.

7 Melt the carob or chocolate in a bowl over a pan of hot water or heat briefly in the microwave. Spread over the surface of the cake and leave to set. Cut into squares before serving.

Tolerant to ...	Variations
➤ Wheat	Use plain (all-purpose) flour.
☺ Eggs	Use 2 beaten eggs instead of the egg replacer and omit 75 ml/5 tbsp of the water.
♥ Dairy	Use butter or ordinary margarine.
☻ Nuts	Add 50 g/2 oz/^{1}/$_2$ cup chopped walnuts to the mixture, if liked.

Fruit Crunchies

Ring the changes by flavouring these with 2.5 ml/½ tsp of ground cinnamon, ginger, mixed spice or the finely grated rind of half a lemon or orange. For US readers, if your child cannot eat corn, avoid light corn syrup and use clear honey instead.

MAKES 20–24

75 g/3 oz/¹⁄₃ cup dairy-free margarine 🥛

75 g/3 oz/¹⁄₃ cup soft light brown sugar

25 ml/1½ tbsp golden (light corn) syrup

5 ml/1 tsp bicarbonate of soda (baking soda)

75 g/3 oz/³⁄₄ cup wheat-free/gluten-free flour mix ✎

100 g/4 oz/1 cup millet flakes 🌾

50 g/2 oz/¹⁄₃ cup dried mixed fruit (fruit cake mix)

1 Melt the margarine, sugar and syrup in a saucepan.

2 Add the bicarbonate of soda – it will froth. Stir in the flour, millet and fruit.

3 Shape into walnut-sized balls and place a little apart on two greased baking (cookie) sheets.

4 Flatten slightly with a fork. Bake in a preheated oven at 190°C/375°F/gas mark 5 (fan oven 170°C) for about 10 minutes until golden. Leave to cool for a few minutes, then transfer to a wire rack to cool completely. Store in an airtight container.

Tolerant to ...	Variations
✎ Wheat	Use plain (all-purpose) or wholemeal flour.
🥛 Dairy	Use butter or ordinary margarine.
🌾 Oats	Use rolled oats instead of millet flakes.

Flapjacks

In the US, if your child is allergic to corn, use clear honey or maple syrup instead of light corn syrup.

MAKES 8 WEDGES

A little oil, for greasing

65 g/2½ oz/scant ⅓ cup dairy-free margarine 🥛

30 ml/2 tbsp granulated sugar

15 ml/1 tbsp golden (light corn) syrup

100 g/4 oz/1 cup millet flakes 🌾

20 g/¾ oz/3 tbsp wheat-free/gluten-free flour mix ✎

1 Lightly grease an 18 cm/7 in non-stick sandwich tin (pan).

2 Melt the margarine, sugar and syrup in a saucepan.

3 Stir in the millet and flour.

4 Press firmly into the prepared tin.

5 Bake in a preheated oven at 180°C/350°F/gas mark 4 (fan oven 160°C) for about 20–25 minutes until golden brown.

6 Leave to cool slightly, then mark into wedges with a knife. When completely cold, cut the wedges and remove from the tin.

Tolerant to ...	Variations
🌾 Oats	Use rolled oats instead of millet flakes, for a change.
✎ Wheat	Use plain (all-purpose) flour.
🥛 Dairy	Use butter or ordinary margarine.

Florentines

---

50 g/2 oz/¹/₄ cup dairy-free margarine 🥛

50 g/2 oz/¹/₄ cup caster (superfine) sugar

50 g/2 oz/¹/₃ cup dried apricots, chopped ☺

3 glacé (candied) cherries, chopped

15 ml/1 tbsp angelica, chopped

15 ml/1 tbsp chopped mixed (candied) peel

15 ml/1 tbsp sultanas (golden raisins)

5 ml/1 tsp dairy-free milk 🥛

15 ml/1 tbsp potato flour ╲

100 g/4 oz/1 cup dairy-free/gluten-free carob or plain (semi-sweet) chocolate, broken up 🥛

---

1 Put the margarine and caster sugar in a saucepan and bring to the boil, stirring.

2 Remove from the heat and stir in all the remaining ingredients except the carob or chocolate. Mix well.

3 Put spoonfuls of the mixture, well apart, on two baking (cookie) sheets, lined with non-stick baking parchment.

4 Bake in a preheated oven at 180°C/350°F/gas mark 4 (fan oven 160°C) for 20 minutes or until golden brown. Leave to cool completely. Loosen and turn over each Florentine.

5 Melt the carob or chocolate in a bowl over a pan of hot water or heat briefly in the microwave. Spoon a little on the flat underside of each Florentine in turn, spreading to cover the base, and leave upside-down to set. Store in an airtight container.

Tolerant to ...	Variations
🥛 Dairy	Use butter or ordinary margarine, cows' milk and any carob or chocolate (check for gluten content, if necessary).
🌰 Nuts	Substitute chopped almonds for the dried apricots, if liked.
🌾 Wheat	Use plain (all-purpose) flour.

Strawberry Chews

These are also delicious made with apricot jam and white marshmallows.

MAKES 16

---

50 g/2 oz/¹/₄ cup dairy-free margarine 🥛

45 ml/3 tbsp strawberry jam (conserve)

50 g/2 oz pink marshmallows

100 g/4 oz/2 cups rice crispies

A few extra marshmallows, for decorating

1 Melt the margarine with the jam and marshmallows in a saucepan, stirring.

2 Stir in the rice crispies and spoon into paper cake cases (cupcake papers). Sprinkle with a few chopped marshmallows. Chill until firm.

Tolerant to ...	Variations
🥛 Dairy	Use butter or ordinary margarine.

Gingerbread Men

If your child likes a stronger ginger taste, you can use up to double the quantity of ginger. These are very crunchy!

MAKES 12

350 g/12 oz/3 cups wheat-free/gluten-free flour mix, plus extra for dusting

1.5 ml/¼ tsp salt

2.5 ml/½ tsp bicarbonate of soda (baking soda)

5 ml/1 tsp ground ginger

1.5 ml/¼ tsp ground cinnamon

50 g/2 oz/¼ cup dairy-free margarine

100 g/4 oz/½ cup soft light brown sugar

30 ml/2 tbsp black treacle (molasses)

45 ml/3 tbsp dairy-free milk

A few currants and glacé (candied) cherries

75 g/3 oz/½ cup icing (confectioners') sugar, sifted

10 ml/2 tsp water

1 Sift the flour, salt, bicarbonate of soda and spices into a bowl.

2 Put the margarine, sugar, treacle and milk in a saucepan and heat gently until the fat melts.

3 Pour into the dry ingredients and mix to form a firm dough. Leave to cool, then chill for 30 minutes.

4 Roll out the dough on a lightly floured surface to about 5 mm/¼ in thick. Cut into 12 shapes using a gingerbread-man cutter. Place well apart on greased baking (cookie) sheets. Press in currants for eyes and buttons and pieces of cherry for mouths.

5 Bake in a preheated oven at 160°C/325°F/gas mark 3 (fan oven 145°C) for 15–20 minutes until firm. Take care not to over-brown the limbs. Cool slightly, then transfer to a wire rack to cool completely.

6 When cold, mix the icing sugar with the water to a smooth cream. Place in a piping bag fitted with a plain tube (tip) or in a paper piping bag with the point snipped off. Pipe bow ties and collars and cuffs on the men. Leave to set. Store in an airtight container.

Tolerant to ...	Variations
Wheat	Use plain (all-purpose) flour.
Dairy	Use butter or ordinary margarine and cows' milk – full-cream for under-5s, semi-skimmed for older children.

Crisp Shorties

MAKES 16

A little oil, for greasing

50 g/2 oz/½ cup rice flour ⬉

50 g/2 oz/½ cup potato flour ⬉ ͡

2.5 ml/½ tsp gluten-free baking powder

50 g/2 oz/¼ cup caster (superfine) sugar

5 ml/1 tsp natural vanilla essence (extract)

75 g/3 oz/⅓ cup dairy-free margarine ⬙

10 glacé (candied) cherries, halved

1   Lightly grease a baking (cookie) sheet.

2   Sift the flours together with the baking powder into a bowl. Stir in the sugar. Add the vanilla essence and margarine and work with a fork until the mixture is blended, then draw together into a ball with your hands.

3   Shape into 16 small balls and place a little apart on the prepared baking (cookie) sheet. Dip the fork in water, then use to flatten each ball of dough. Press half a glacé cherry in the centre of each biscuit (cookie).

4   Bake in a preheated oven at 180°C/350°F/gas mark 4 (fan oven 160°C) for 20–25 minutes until golden brown.

5   Remove from the oven. Leave to cool for 10 minutes then transfer to a wire rack to cool completely. Store in an airtight container.

Tolerant to ...	Variations
⬙ Dairy	Use butter or ordinary margarine.
͡ Soya	Substitute soya flour for the potato flour.
⬉ Wheat	Use plain (all-purpose) flour instead of the rice and potato flours.

Pancakes

100 g/4 oz/1 cup buckwheat flour ✎

1.5 ml/¼ tsp salt

5 ml/1 tsp No Egg egg replacer (see page 20) ◯

30 ml/2 tbsp warm water

300 ml/½ pt/1¼ cups dairy-free milk 🍶

60 ml/4 tbsp cold water

45 ml/3 tbsp sunflower oil, plus extra for cooking

1 Mix the flour and salt in a bowl.

2 Whisk the egg replacer and warm water together until frothy. Add to the flour with half the milk and beat well. Stir in the remaining milk, the cold water and the measured oil.

3 Heat a little oil in a small frying pan (skillet). Pour off the excess.

4 Add a large spoonful of the batter and quickly swirl round the pan to coat the base. Cook until holes appear on the surface and the pancake is golden brown underneath.

5 Flip the pancake over and cook the other side briefly until browned. Slide on to a plate and keep warm over a pan of hot water while cooking the rest. Serve hot.

Tolerant to ...	Variations
✎ Wheat	Use plain (all-purpose) or wholemeal flour.
◯ Eggs	Use 1 egg instead of the egg replacer and omit the warm water. Add to the flour, then continue as above, omitting the cold water as well.
🍶 Dairy	Use cows' milk – full-cream for under-5s, semi-skimmed for older children.

Savoury Light Pancakes

These egg-free pancakes are perfect for serving with any filling or sauce of your choice. To make Sweet Light Pancakes, use grated sweet potato instead of ordinary potato. The wheat, dairy and egg options are the same.

MAKES ABOUT 8

---

75 g/3 oz potatoes, peeled and grated ⟁

100 g/4 oz/1 cup wheat-free/gluten-free flour mix ⟍

10 ml/2 tsp gluten-free baking powder

A good pinch of salt

30 ml/2 tbsp sunflower oil, plus extra for cooking

300 ml/½ pt/1¼ cups dairy-free milk ⛟

---

1 Mix all the ingredients together in a bowl and beat until smooth.

2 Heat a little oil in a small frying pan (skillet) until very hot. Pour off the excess.

3 Add a large spoonful of the batter to the pan and swirl to coat the base of the pan. Cook over a moderate heat for 2–3 minutes (little bubbles will appear and burst on the surface) until golden underneath and set on top.

4 Turn over and cook the other side until golden. Slide out of the pan and keep warm. Repeat until all the batter is used, stirring the batter thoroughly before making each pancake. Use as required.

Tolerant to ...	Variations
⟍ Wheat	Use plain (all-purpose) flour.
⛟ Dairy	Use cows' milk – full-cream for under-5s, semi-skimmed for older children.
⟁ Eggs	Use 1 egg instead of the potato.

Yorkshire Puddings

You need the gum to get a proper 'rise'. Use guar gum if your child is allergic to corn.

MAKES 12

Sunflower oil, for cooking

100 g/4 oz/1 cup wheat-free/gluten-free flour mix ❋

5 ml/1 tsp xanthum gum

15 ml/1 tbsp gluten-free baking powder

A good pinch of salt

75 g/3 oz potatoes, peeled and grated ⊙

150 ml/¼ pt/⅔ cup dairy-free milk 🖠

150 ml/¼ pt/⅔ cup water

---

1 Preheat the oven at 200°C/400°F/gas mark 6 (fan oven 180°C). Put a little oil in 12 sections of a tartlet tin (patty pan) and place in the oven.

2 Sift the flour, gum, baking powder and salt into a bowl.

3 Add the grated potato and half the milk and water. Beat well until blended. Stir in the remaining milk and water.

4 When the oil is sizzling hot, spoon the batter into the sections of the tin. Cook towards the top of the oven for 25 minutes until risen, crisp and golden.

Tolerant to ...	Variations
❋ Wheat	Use plain (all-purpose) flour instead of the wheat-free/gluten-free mix and omit the xanthum gum.
🖠 Dairy	Use cows' milk – full-cream for under-5s, semi-skimmed for older children.
⊙ Eggs	Use 1 large egg and omit the potato.

SWEETS, TREATS AND PARTY SPECIALS

Parties can be a nightmare if your child has food allergies or intolerances. Everything you would normally serve, from sandwiches to cakes to sausage rolls, contains wheat, gluten, dairy products and, probably, eggs. You cannot be sure that bought foods don't contain traces of nuts either. So in this section I've created a whole spread of party foods that even children without allergies will tuck into with delight. There is also a range of sweets and treats because many chocolates and candies have to be avoided by allergenic children. If your children want to help make them, do be careful: sugar has to be heated to very high temperatures to make sweets and can cause serious burns. Never let your child make them unsupervised.

CRISPS AND CHOCOLATE

Take care when buying crisps (potato chips). Many flavoured ones contain potential allergens. Note, too, that the potato 'snacks' in cardboard tubes may contain wheat starch (although they may be gluten-free).

Many of the large supermarkets and health food shops sell plain (semi-sweet) chocolate that is free from dairy products. Look for the luxury Belgian, Fair-trade and Organic brands with a high cocoa butter content. Beware, however, if your child is allergic to soya – many contain soya lecithin.

Tortilla Chips

You can flavour these with onion or garlic salt, or add a pinch of chilli powder for extra zing. Serve them with a Fresh Tomato Salsa (see page 170) or Avocado Dip (see page 171) for a tasty treat. If your child is allergic to corn, use the all-flour version of the tortillas.

SERVES 6–8

1 quantity of Tortillas (see page 127)

Sunflower oil, for cooking

1.5 ml/¼ tsp celery salt

1 Cut each tortilla into six wedges.

2 Heat about 5 mm/¼ in of oil in a frying pan (skillet).

3 Add a few wedges at a time and cook, turning once or twice, until golden and crisp.

4 Drain on kitchen paper (paper towels). Repeat with the remaining wedges. Leave to cool.

5 Place the chips in a bowl, sprinkle with the flavoured salt and toss gently to coat.

Pizza Faces

If your child is allergic to tomatoes, simply omit the tomato purée. For added flavour, in that case, spread with Brown Table Sauce (see page 166), if liked. You can top the pizzas with soya, buffalo Mozzarella or hard sheep's cheese, if your child can tolerate them.

MAKES 8

---

1 large potato, scrubbed

25 g/1 oz/2 tbsp dairy-free margarine 🥛

75 g/3 oz/¾ cup rice flour, plus a little for dusting

2.5 ml/½ tsp gluten-free baking powder

A good pinch of salt

10–15 ml/½–1 tbsp dairy-free milk 🥛

30 ml/2 tbsp sunflower or olive oil

30 ml/2 tbsp tomato purée (paste)

2.5 ml/½ tsp dried oregano

75 g/3 oz/¾ cup grated No-allergen Hard Cheese (see page 178) 🥛

1 small carrot, coarsely grated

4 stuffed olives

Pieces of green and red (bell) pepper, for decorating

---

1 Prick the potato and cook in the microwave for about 4 minutes until soft, then remove the skin. Alternatively, peel, cut into chunks and boil in water until tender, then drain.

2 Mash well in a bowl with the margarine and work in the flour, baking powder, salt and enough milk to form a firm dough.

3   Dust a surface with rice flour and roll out the dough to about 5 mm/¼ in thick. Using a 7.5 cm/3 in cutter, cut into eight rounds, re-kneading and rolling the dough as necessary.

4   Heat the oil in a large frying pan (skillet) and add the potato rounds. Cook for about 2 minutes until the bases are golden brown. Turn over. You may need to do this in two batches.

5   Spread with the tomato purée, then top with the oregano, then the cheese. Arrange the grated carrot round the top half of each pizza, to look like hair. Slice each olive into four, to make round 'eyes'. Cut diamond shapes from the green pepper for noses and slices from the red pepper for lips. Add to the pizza faces.

6   Cover the pan(s) with lids or foil and cook over a fairly gentle heat for about 3 minutes or until the cheese has melted. Serve hot or cold.

Tolerant to ...	Variations
Dairy	Use butter or ordinary margarine and cows' milk. Top with Cheddar cheese or Mozzarella if you prefer.
Wheat	Use plain (all-purpose) flour.

Mini Quiches

*These bite-sized morsels are popular with most children –
with or without allergies! Use other fillings for a change, such
as sliced mushrooms, drained canned sweetcorn, chopped
tomatoes or peppers.*

MAKES 12

---

*⅓ quantity of Dairy-free/Gluten-free Savoury Pastry
(see page 165)*

Rice flour, for dusting

75 g/3 oz streaky bacon, rinded and diced

30 ml/2 tbsp No Egg egg replacer (see page 20)

150 ml/¼ pt/⅔ cup hot dairy-free milk

Salt and freshly ground black pepper

2.5 ml/½ tsp dried mixed herbs

1 Roll out the pastry (paste) on a surface dusted with rice
   flour. Cut into 12 rounds using a 7.5 cm/3 in biscuit
   (cookie) cutter.

2 Press into the greased sections of a tartlet tin (patty
   pan). Bake in a preheated oven at 200°C/400°F/gas
   mark 6 (fan oven 180°C) for 5 minutes to part-cook.

3 Dry-fry the bacon, stirring all the time, until cooked
   and the fat runs. Drain on kitchen paper (paper
   towels).

4 Whisk the egg replacer with the hot milk, a little salt
   and pepper and the herbs.

5 Spoon the bacon into the pastry cases (pie shells).
   Spoon the milk mixture over. Bake in the oven for a
   further 12–15 minutes until golden and set. Cool
   slightly, then remove from the tin and serve warm or
   cold.

Tolerant to ...	Variations
❀ Wheat	Make up your ordinary shortcrust pastry (basic pie crust) recipe, using half white vegetable fat and half dairy-free margarine, if necessary. Use plain (all-purpose) flour.
☙ Dairy	Use butter or ordinary margarine in the pastry. Use cows' milk – full-cream for under-5s, semi-skimmed for older children.
☺ Eggs	Use 1 beaten egg instead of the egg replacer and reduce the milk by 30 ml/2 tbsp.

Stuffed Cherry Tomatoes

You can also use soft soya, sheep's or goats' cheese, if your child can tolerate them.

MAKES 24

24 cherry tomatoes

225 g/8 oz/1 cup Non-dairy Soft Cheese (see page 180) ☙ ✖

15 ml/1 tbsp Sweet Brown Pickle (see page 168) ❀

1 Cut a slice off the rounded end of each tomato and scoop out the seeds. Drain upside-down on kitchen paper (paper towels).

2 Mix the cheese with the pickle. Spoon into the tomatoes. Rest the slices on tops as 'lids'. Arrange on a serving plate and chill until ready to serve.

Tolerant to ...	Variations
☙ Dairy	Use ordinary soft white cheese, such as Philadelphia, or cheese spread.
❀ Wheat	Use ordinary sweet pickle.
✖ Fish	Use an 85 g/3½ oz/very small can of tuna, drained and mashed, instead of half the cheese, if liked.

Crunchy Garbanzos

Make these when the oven is on for something else. They can be cooked at the bottom of a slightly hotter oven or at the top of a slightly cooler one, if necessary.

SERVES 8

2 × 425 g/15 oz/large cans of chick peas (garbanzos), drained

10 ml/2 tsp garam masala

5 ml/1 tsp ground cumin

A good pinch of salt

1 Dry the chick peas on kitchen paper (paper towels), then toss in the spices and salt.

2 Spread out on a baking (cookie) sheet and bake in a preheated oven at 180°C/350°F/gas mark 4 (fan oven 160°C) for about 1 hour until brown and crisp, stirring around once halfway through cooking. Cool, then store in an airtight container.

Crispy Potato Skins

When preparing potatoes for a meal, scrub them before peeling, then use the skins for this tasty and nutritious snack. Obviously, the quantities don't matter.

Scrubbed potato peelings

Salt

1 Spread the potato peelings in a thin even layer on a baking (cookie) sheet. Sprinkle lightly with salt.

2 Bake in a preheated oven at 200°C/400°F/gas mark 6 (fan oven 180°C) for about 20 minutes or until crisp and golden. Cool, then store in an airtight container.

Sausage Rolls

MAKES 32 ROLLS

1 quantity of Dairy-free/Gluten-free Savoury Pastry (see page 165) `⬎`

A little rice flour, for dusting `⬎`

1 quantity of sausagemeat (see page 51)

Dairy-free milk, for glazing `⬆` `⌒`

1 Cut the pastry (paste) into four pieces. Dust a surface with rice flour. Roll out each piece to an oblong about 10 cm/4 in wide.

2 Cut the sausagemeat into four and shape each piece into a sausage as long as the pastry oblongs. Lay one sausage to the side of each oblong.

3 Brush the edges of the pastry with milk, then fold over the sausagemeat and press the long edges together to seal. Knock up the sealed edges with the back of a knife, then make several small slashes diagonally across the length of the top to decorate. Cut each one into eight small sausage rolls.

4 Transfer to lightly greased baking (cookie) sheets and brush with a little milk to glaze. Bake in a preheated oven at 200°C/400°F/gas mark 6 (fan oven 180°C) for about 20–25 minutes until golden and cooked through. Serve warm or cold.

Tolerant to ...	Variations
`⬎` Wheat	Make up your ordinary shortcrust pastry (basic pie crust) recipe, using half white vegetable fat and half dairy-free margarine, if necessary. Use plain (all-purpose) flour for dusting.
`⬆` Dairy	Use butter or ordinary margarine in the pastry and cows' milk for glazing.
`⌒` Eggs	Use beaten egg to glaze the sausage rolls instead of milk, if you prefer.

Mallow Fudge

For a change, add 50 g/2 oz/¹/₃ cup raisins and flavour with rum essence instead of the vanilla.

MAKES 36 PIECES

100 g/4 oz/1 small packet of marshmallows

30 ml/2 tbsp dairy-free milk 🥛

50 g/2 oz/¹/₄ cup soft light brown sugar

50 g/2 oz/¹/₄ cup dairy-free margarine 🥛

100 g/4 oz/²/₃ cup icing (confectioners') sugar, sifted

5 ml/1 tsp natural vanilla essence (extract)

1 Put the marshmallows in a saucepan with half the milk. Heat gently until the marshmallows melt. Remove from the heat.

2 In a separate pan, put the brown sugar and margarine and heat until melted. Bring to the boil and boil for 5 minutes.

3 Remove from the heat and stir in the marshmallows, icing sugar, remaining milk and the vanilla essence. Mix thoroughly.

4 Spread in an oiled 18 cm/7 in square, shallow baking tin (pan). Leave until cold and set. Cut into squares.

Tolerant to ...	Variations
🥜 Nuts	Add 50 g/2 oz/¹/₂ cup chopped mixed nuts, if liked.
🥛 Dairy	Use butter or ordinary margarine and cows' milk.

Toffee Apples

I use 5 mm/¹/₄ in dowelling, cut into 15 cm/6 in lengths, for the sticks, but you could improvise with wooden chopsticks. It is important that the toffee is at the right temperature or it won't stick to the apples.

MAKES 8

8 small eating (dessert) apples

450 g/1 lb/2 cups demerara sugar

50 g/2 oz/¹/₄ cup dairy-free margarine 🛢

15 ml/1 tbsp white wine vinegar

150 ml/¹/₄ pt/²/₃ cup water

1 Scrub the apples and dry on kitchen paper (paper towels). Push a stick into each core to hold the fruit firmly.

2 Put the remaining ingredients in a heavy-based saucepan. Melt very slowly over a gentle heat until the sugar has completely dissolved, stirring occasionally.

3 When it has dissolved, bring to the boil and boil to 122°C/252°F on a sugar thermometer or until the mixture has turned a deep golden brown and a small spoonful forms a hard ball when dropped into a cup of cold water.

4 Quickly dip the apples in the hot toffee to coat completely, twirl round for a few seconds, then transfer to non-stick baking parchment on a baking (cookie) sheet to set.

Tolerant to ...	Variations
🛢 Dairy	Use butter or ordinary margarine.

Jam Sandwich Biscuits

If your child is allergic to corn, use arrowroot
instead of cornflour.

MAKES 14

100g/4 oz/1 cup cornflour (cornstarch)

100 g/4 oz/1 cup rice flour ✎

200 g/7 oz/generous 1 cup icing (confectioners') sugar

225 g/8 oz/1 cup dairy-free margarine 🍶

45 ml/3 tbsp seedless raspberry jam (clear conserve)

2.5 ml/¹/₂ tsp natural vanilla essence (extract)

1 Sift the flours and 75 g/3 oz/¹/₂ cup of the icing sugar together in a bowl. Add 175 g/6 oz/³/₄ cup of the margarine and work in with a fork to form a dough. Wrap in foil or clingfilm (plastic wrap) and chill for 30 minutes.

2 Roll out the dough fairly thinly and cut into 28 rounds, using a 6 cm/2¹/₂ in cutter. Place a little apart on baking (cookie) sheets, lined with non-stick baking parchment.

3 Use the end of a wooden spoon to make a small hole through the centre of half the biscuits (cookies). Spoon a little raspberry jam into each hole.

4 Bake in a preheated oven at 160°C/325°F/gas mark 3 (fan oven 145°C) for 20–25 minutes until lightly golden.

5 Leave to cool on the baking sheets.

6 Meanwhile, sift the remaining icing sugar and work in the remaining margarine and the vanilla essence.

7 Spread this mixture on the underside of the plain biscuits. Carefully lift the jam-filled biscuits off the paper and place on top. Store in an airtight container.

Tolerant to ...	Variations
❤ Dairy	Use butter instead of the dairy-free margarine.
❦ Wheat	Use plain (all-purpose) flour instead of the rice flour.

Buttery-crisp Popcorn

If your child is allergic to corn, try making tiny clusters of Buttery-crisp Pop Rice. Melt the syrup (US readers should use clear honey, not light corn syrup) with the margarine until bubbling, stir in rice crispies until coated, then drop the mixture in tiny clusters on a lightly oiled baking (cookie) sheet to set.

MAKES 1 LARGE BOWL

40 g/1½ oz/3 tbsp dairy-free margarine ❤

50 g/2 oz/½ cup popping corn (maize)

45 ml/3 tbsp golden (light corn) syrup

1 Melt 25 g/1 oz/2 tbsp of the margarine in a large non-stick saucepan with a lid.

2 Add the corn, cover, shake the pan vigorously and cook over a moderate heat. The corn will start to pop. Hold the lid on firmly and shake the pan from time to time until all the popping stops.

3 Remove the lid and stir in the remaining margarine and the syrup, over a gentle heat, stirring all the time for 3–4 minutes until each piece of corn is coated stickily and the mixture is hot but not burning.

4 Tip into a large bowl and leave to cool. Store any leftovers in an airtight container.

Tolerant to ...	Variations
❤ Dairy	Use butter or ordinary margarine.

Toffee Krispies

In the US, if your child is allergic to corn, use maple syrup or clear honey instead of light corn syrup.

MAKES 24

A little oil, for greasing

50 g/2 oz/¼ cup dairy-free margarine 🥛

100 g/4 oz/1 small packet of marshmallows

30 ml/2 tbsp golden (light corn) syrup

150 g/5 oz/2½ cups rice crispies

1 Oil an 18 × 28 cm/7 × 11 in Swiss roll tin (jelly roll pan).

2 Put the margarine, marshmallows and syrup in a heavy-based saucepan and heat gently, stirring until melted. Stir in the cereal.

3 Press the mixture into the tin, using the back of a wet spoon.

4 Leave until cold and set firm. Cut into squares.

Tolerant to ...	Variations
🥛 Dairy	Use butter or ordinary margarine.

Banana and Rose-hip Smoothie

SERVES 1

1 ripe banana

10 ml/2 tsp rose-hip syrup

200 ml/7 fl oz/scant 1 cup dairy-free milk 🥛

A pinch of ground cinnamon

1 Break the banana into pieces and put in a blender or food processor. Add the remaining ingredients.

2 Run the machine until thick and frothy. Pour into a glass and serve immediately.

Tolerant to ...	Variations
🥛 Dairy	Use cows' milk – full-cream for under-5s, semi-skimmed for older children.

Carob or Chocolate Smoothie

The avocado gives a thick, nutritious richness without altering the flavour. As an alternative, use a banana. For an extra treat, float a scoop of vanilla dairy-free ice cream on top before serving.

SERVES 1

½ small ripe avocado, halved and stoned (pitted)

15 ml/1 tbsp clear honey

15 ml/1 tbsp pure carob or cocoa (unsweetened chocolate) powder

A few drops of natural vanilla essence (extract)

200 ml/7 fl oz/scant 1 cup dairy-free milk, chilled 🥛

1 Scoop the avocado flesh into a blender or food processor. Add the honey and blend briefly until smooth.

2 Add the remaining ingredients and run the machine until thick and frothy. Serve straight away.

Tolerant to ...	Variations
🥛 Dairy	Use cows' milk – full-cream for under-5s, semi-skimmed for older children.

Happy Face Cakes

MAKES 12

---

1 quantity of Vanilla Sponge Cake mix (see page 130)

50 g/2 oz/¹/₄ cup dairy-free margarine 🥛

150 g/5 oz/scant 1 cup icing (confectioners') sugar, sifted

A few drops of natural vanilla essence (extract)

24 currants or dried blueberries

6 glacé (candied) cherries

3 squares of dairy-free/gluten-free carob or plain (semi-sweet) chocolate, coarsely grated ⬉

---

1 Make up the cake mixture and spoon into 12 paper cake cases (cupcake papers) in a tartlet tin (patty pan).

2 Bake in a preheated oven at 180°C/350°F/gas mark 4 (fan oven 160°C) for about 18 minutes until the cakes are risen and golden and the centres spring back when pressed.

3 Transfer to a wire rack to cool.

4 Blend the margarine with the icing sugar and vanilla essence. Spread over the tops of the cold cakes.

5 Use the currants or blueberries for eyes. Cut pieces of cherry for noses and mouths and add the grated carob or chocolate for hair.

Tolerant to ...	Variations
🥛 Dairy	Use softened butter instead of the dairy-free margarine.
⬉ Wheat	Use liquorice bootlaces for mouths and/or hair or to make animal faces with ears and whiskers, if liked.

PASTRIES, CONDIMENTS AND ACCOMPANIMENTS

There are so many extra things that children with allergies or intolerances often can't enjoy – brown table sauce, sweet pickle, mayonnaise and even dill pickles. This section includes allergen-free versions of all of these, plus other sauces and relishes, non-dairy cheeses, milks and creams, a few speciality spreads, a wheat-free/gluten-free flour mix and all the odds and ends that don't fit anywhere else! Note that I have included a Nut Milk and a Nut Cream – these are, quite obviously, unsuitable for anyone with a nut allergy, but they are so good for children who can't tolerate dairy products, I simply had to include them.

I used to make my own non-dairy cheeses with tofu, but now that there is such a good range of soya cheeses on the market, it's not worth it. However, if your child can't eat dairy products or soya, don't worry, I've discovered how to make a brilliant hard cheese substitute (see page 178) that doesn't contain any animal or vegetable allergens. I've also made a non-dairy soft cheese (see page 180) with sheep's yoghurt, which tastes very similar to Philadelphia.

PICKLES

You'd think that pickled onions or dill pickles would be fine for everyone, but it's not so. Most pickles and chutneys are made with malt vinegar (either brown or distilled white) and the malt usually comes from barley, which contains gluten. Also, many thick pickles and chutneys contain wheat flour and some may contain dairy products in the form of lactose or casein in some form or another. And, if they don't contain any of these, soya may well feature in the ingredients list. So, once again, the bottom line is, always read the labels!

Wheat-free/Gluten-free Flour Mix

You can buy commercially made wheat-free/gluten-free flour mix but making it yourself is much cheaper. Unfortunately it doesn't work quite like ordinary wheat flour, because it's the gluten in wheat that makes it elastic. You can make the flour mix more like ordinary flour for use in your own recipes by adding 5 ml/1 tsp of xanthum gum (or guar gum if your child is allergic to corn) to every 100 g/4 oz/1 cup of flour mix. The gum makes the flour more elastic. You will also need to make the mixture wetter than with conventional flour, so you will need to experiment a bit – it isn't as straighforward as it sounds!

In the recipe below, I have used buckwheat flour because it is readily available but it does have a distinctive taste, so you may prefer to bulk-buy tapioca flour by mail order (see page 186) and use that in place of the buckwheat.

If your child is allergic to corn, omit the cornflour and use an extra 50 g/2 oz/¹/₂ cup of buckwheat (or tapioca) flour.

You can also buy gluten-free white bread flour with gum already added. I have used this mix for the soft white bread recipe on page 122. I found that it wasn't suitable for ordinary baking, though – it is too 'gluey'.

MAKES 700 G/1¹/₂ LB/6 CUPS
50 g/2 oz/¹/₂ cup buckwheat flour
50 g/2 oz/¹/₂ cup cornflour (cornstarch)
100 g/4 oz/1 cup potato flour
450 g/1 lb/4 cups white rice flour

Sift all the flours together and store in an airtight container.

Dairy-free/Gluten-free Savoury Pastry

It's not worth making less than this quantity, but you can freeze it. However, it becomes a little moist on thawing. To rectify this, simply knead in a little rice flour before using.

MAKES ABOUT 700 G/1½ LB

450 g/1 lb potatoes, scrubbed and cut into pieces ↖

100 g/4 oz/½ cup dairy-free margarine 🥛

175 g/6 oz/1½ cups rice flour, plus extra for dusting ↖

5 ml/1 tsp salt

1 Cook the potatoes in plenty of boiling water until tender. Drain.

2 Peel off the skins and mash the potatoes well with the margarine.

3 Add the flour and salt and work together to form a dough. Wrap in a plastic bag and chill for 1 hour.

4 Roll out on a surface dusted with rice flour and use as required.

Tolerant to ...	Variations
↖ Wheat	Make shortcrust pastry (basic pie crust) using your usual recipe but use half white vegetable fat and half dairy-free margarine, if necessary. Use plain (all-purpose) flour for dusting.
🥛 Dairy	Use butter or ordinary margarine.

Dairy-free/Gluten-free Sweet Pastry

MAKES ABOUT 700 G/1½ LB

Prepare exactly as Dairy-free/Gluten-free Savoury Pastry but use sweet potatoes or yams instead of ordinary potatoes and omit the salt. For wheat variation, use a sweet pastry (paste) recipe.

Brown Table Sauce

For a slightly sharper, hotter sauce (like the HP original), add an extra 15–30 ml/1–2 tbsp of white wine vinegar blended with 2.5 ml/½ tsp of potato flour and a generous dash of Tabasco.

MAKES ABOUT 350 ML/12 FL OZ/1⅓ CUPS

1 onion, roughly chopped

100 g/4 oz/⅔ cup dried stoned (pitted) dates

1 small eating (dessert) apple, peeled, cored and roughly chopped

25 g/1 oz/1½ tbsp tamarind pulp

150 ml/¼ pt/⅔ cup balsamic vinegar

150 ml/¼ pt/⅔ cup water

10 ml/2 tsp black treacle (molasses)

5 ml/1 tsp soft light brown sugar

1.5 ml/¼ tsp ground allspice

5 ml/1 tsp salt

Freshly ground black pepper

5 ml/1 tsp potato flour

45 ml/3 tbsp white wine vinegar

A few drops of Tabasco sauce

1 Put all the ingredients except the potato flour, white wine vinegar and Tabasco in a saucepan. Bring to the boil, reduce the heat, cover and simmer very gently for 20 minutes until pulpy.

2 Check there are no large tamarind seeds in the mixture – remove any you find. Tip the mixture into a blender or food processor and run the machine until smooth.

3 Rub the mixture through a sieve (strainer), back into the saucepan. Blend the potato flour with the white wine vinegar. Stir into the mixture, bring to the boil and simmer for 2 minutes. Season to taste with Tabasco and more salt and pepper, if necessary. Leave until cold. Pour into a screw-topped container and use as required.

Barbecue Dipping Sauce

This can also be used to coat chicken pieces or pork chops before grilling. Pimenton is a sweet red pepper with a lovely smoky flavour.

SERVES 4

60 ml/4 tbsp gluten-free tomato ketchup (catsup)

30 ml/2 tbsp clear honey

15 ml/1 tbsp gluten-free Worcestershire sauce

15 ml/1 tbsp red wine vinegar

1.5 ml/¼ tsp ground pimenton

Mix all the ingredients together until well blended. Use as required.

Sweet Brown Pickle

I use a mixture of marrow, onions, beans, cucumber and cauliflower for this recipe. The vegetables should be weighed after preparation.

MAKES ABOUT 900 G/2 LB

900 g/2 lb chopped mixed vegetables

100 g/4 oz/1 cup salt

100 g/4 oz/¹/₂ cup soft dark brown sugar

100 g/4 oz/²/₃ cup dates, stoned (pitted) and chopped

5 ml/1 tsp gluten-free mustard powder

2.5 ml/¹/₂ tsp ground ginger

2.5 ml/¹/₂ tsp ground allspice

450 ml/³/₄ pt/2 cups white wine vinegar

150 ml/¹/₄ pt/²/₃ cup water

150 ml/¹/₄ pt/²/₃ cup balsamic vinegar

20 ml/1¹/₂ tbsp potato flour

Garlic salt

Freshly ground black pepper

1 Layer the vegetables in a large bowl, sprinkling the salt between the layers. Leave to stand for 2 hours. Cover with cold water, stir well, drain, rinse thoroughly with more cold water and drain again.

2 Put the vegetables in a large saucepan or preserving pan with the sugar, dates, mustard, ginger, allspice, white wine vinegar and water. Bring to the boil, reduce the heat, part-cover and simmer gently for about 10 minutes until the vegetables are cooked but still have some 'bite'.

3 Blend the balsamic vinegar with the potato flour and stir into the pickle. Bring back to the boil and cook for 2 minutes, stirring until thick. Taste and add a little garlic salt and pepper, if liked.

4 Spoon the pickle into clean, warm jars. Cover, label, leave until cold, then store in a cool, dark place.

Dill-pickled Cucumber Slices

SERVES ABOUT 8

½ cucumber

150 ml/¼ pt/⅔ cup white wine vinegar

5 ml/1 tsp dried dill (dill weed)

15 ml/1 tbsp caster (superfine) sugar

6 black peppercorns

1 Cut the cucumber into slices about 3 mm/⅛ in thick. Place in a saucepan.

2 Add the remaining ingredients. Bring to the boil, cover and boil for 1 minute. Leave to cool in the saucepan.

3 Place in a clean, screw-topped jar or other sealable container and store in the fridge for up to 1 month.

Fresh Tomato Salsa

If your children like spicy foods, add a small red chilli, seeded and finely chopped.

SERVES 4

---

4 ripe tomatoes, skinned

200 g/7 oz/1 small can of pimientos, drained

15 ml/1 tbsp tomato purée (paste)

15 ml/1 tbsp red wine vinegar

5 ml/1 tsp soft light brown sugar

Salt and freshly ground black pepper

Put all the ingredients except the salt and pepper in a blender or food processor and run the machine until smooth. Season to taste. Use as required.

Fresh Cucumber Salsa

SERVES 4

¼ cucumber, very finely chopped

2 spring onions (scallions) or ½ small onion, very finely chopped

5 ml/1 tsp dried mint

15 ml/1 tbsp caster (superfine) sugar

15 ml/1 tbsp white wine vinegar

Salt and freshly ground black pepper

Mix all the ingredients in a bowl with seasoning to taste. Leave to stand for at least 1 hour before serving, if possible, to allow the flavours to develop.

Avocado Dip

*This is tasty served with sticks of raw vegetables or my
Tortilla Chips (see page 149), as a party snack or light meal.
It also makes a good sandwich spread or you can serve it as
a relish with grilled meats or fish. Use white wine
vinegar instead of the lemon juice if your child is allergic
to citrus fruit.*

SERVES 4–6

---

2 ripe avocados

1 small piece of onion, grated

15 ml/1 tbsp lemon juice

60 ml/4 tbsp sunflower oil

5 cm/2 in piece of cucumber, finely chopped

½ small red (bell) pepper, finely chopped (optional)

Salt and freshly ground black pepper

A few drops of Tabasco (optional)

1 Halve the avocados and remove the stones (pits).
   Scoop the flesh into a bowl and mash thoroughly with
   a fork.

2 Using a small wire whisk, work in the onion and lemon
   juice. Whisk in the oil, a drop at a time, until thick, like
   mayonnaise.

3 Stir in the cucumber and red pepper, if using. Season to
   taste and add the Tabasco, if using. Spoon the dip into
   a small bowl and chill until ready to serve.

Cool Coleslaw

MAKES ABOUT 350 G/12 OZ

¹/₄ small white cabbage

1 carrot

¹/₄ small onion

60 ml/4 tbsp Egg-free Mayonnaise (see page 177) ⊂⊃

10 ml/2 tsp white wine vinegar

15 ml/1 tbsp sunflower oil

Salt and freshly ground black pepper

A good pinch of caster (superfine) sugar

1   Finely shred or coarsely grate the cabbage and place in a bowl. Coarsely grate the carrot and add to the bowl. Grate the onion and add to the bowl.

2   Add the remaining ingredients to the vegetables, season to taste and mix well. Store in an airtight container in the fridge and use within 3 days.

Tolerant to ...	Variations
⊂⊃ Eggs	Use ordinary mayonnaise.

Savoury White Sauce

You can use this recipe to make Béchamel Sauce, which has more flavour. Put the milk in a saucepan with a bay leaf and slice of onion. Bring to the boil, remove from the heat and infuse until cold. Strain and then make the sauce as below.

SERVES 4

20 g/³⁄₄ oz/3 tbsp cornflour (cornstarch) or rice flour ❧

300 ml/¹⁄₂ pt/1¹⁄₄ cups dairy-free milk 🍶

A good knob of dairy-free margarine 🍶

Salt and freshly ground black pepper

1 Blend the cornflour or rice flour with a little of the milk in a saucepan and stir in the remaining milk.

2 Add the margarine, bring to the boil and cook, stirring, for 1 minute until thickened. Season the sauce to taste and use as required.

Tolerant to ...	Variations
🍶 Dairy	Use cows' milk – full-cream for under-5s, semi-skimmed milk for older children and butter or ordinary margarine.
❧ Wheat	Use plain (all-purpose) flour.

Cheese Sauce

You can use hard soya, sheep's or goats' cheese if your child can tolerate them.

SERVES 4

20 g/³/₄ oz/3 tbsp cornflour (cornstarch) or rice flour ↘

1.5 ml/¹/₄ tsp gluten-free mustard powder

300 ml/¹/₂ pt/1¹/₄ cups dairy-free milk ⊌

A good knob of dairy-free margarine ⊌

50 g/2 oz/¹/₂ cup grated No-allergen Hard Cheese (see page 178) ⊌

Salt and freshly ground black pepper

1 Blend the cornflour or rice flour and mustard with a little of the milk in a saucepan. Stir in the remaining milk and add the margarine.

2 Bring to the boil and cook, stirring, for 1 minute until thickened.

3 Stir in the hard cheese until melted. Season to taste.

Tolerant to ...	Variations
↘ Wheat	Use plain (all-purpose) flour.
⊌ Dairy	Use cows' milk – full-cream for under-5s, semi-skimmed for older children – plus butter or ordinary margarine and Cheddar cheese.

Red Lentil Sauce

This is a useful and nourishing alternative to tomato sauce to serve with pasta, rice, meat, fish or poultry. It can also be spread on pizza bases instead of tomato purée.
Use white wine vinegar instead of lemon juice if your child can't tolerate citrus fruits.

MAKES ABOUT 900 ML/1½ PTS/3¾ CUPS

225 g/8 oz/1⅓ cups red lentils

300 ml/½ pt/1¼ cups water

300 ml/½ pt/1¼ cups apple juice

5 ml/1 tsp dried onion granules

15 ml/1 tbsp lemon juice

1 red (bell) pepper, finely chopped

Salt and freshly ground black pepper

1 Put all the ingredients except the salt and pepper in a saucepan. Bring to the boil, reduce the heat, part-cover and simmer gently for 15 minutes or until tender and most of the liquid has been absorbed.

2 Tip the mixture into a blender or food processor and blend until smooth. Thin, if necessary, to the desired consistency with a little extra apple juice, then season to taste. Either reheat and use straight away or cool, then store in an airtight container in the fridge. Use within 3 days.

Wheat-free/Gluten-free Gravy

This can be served with any savoury meal that needs gravy.

SERVES 4

1 onion, finely chopped

1 carrot, finely chopped

15 g/¹/₂ oz/1 tbsp dairy-free margarine ▮

5 ml/1 tsp soft dark brown sugar

300 ml/¹/₂ pt/1¹/₄ cups vegetable stock, made with 1 dairy-free/gluten-free stock cube

30 ml/2 tbsp cornflour (cornstarch) or rice flour

30 ml/2 tbsp water

Salt and freshly ground black pepper

1 Fry (sauté) the onion and carrot in the margarine, stirring, for 2 minutes. Add the sugar and continue to fry, stirring, for about 5 minutes until it is a deep, rich brown (don't allow it to burn).

2 Stir in the stock, bring to the boil, reduce the heat and simmer for 10 minutes. For smooth gravy, strain the liquid, then return it to the saucepan.

3 Blend the cornflour with the water and stir into the gravy. Bring to the boil and cook for 1 minute, stirring. Season to taste and serve.

Tolerant to ...	Variations
▮ Dairy	Use butter or ordinary margarine.

Egg-free Mayonnaise

You can flavour this with garlic or herbs like any other mayonnaise. For a sharper flavour, add a dash more white wine vinegar. If your child is allergic to citrus fruits, use extra white wine vinegar instead of the lemon juice.

MAKES ABOUT 300 ML/¹⁄₂ PT/1¹⁄₄ CUPS

10 ml/2 tsp potato flour

10 ml/2 tsp arrowroot

2.5 ml/¹⁄₂ tsp caster (superfine) sugar

2.5 ml/¹⁄₂ tsp salt

A good pinch of white pepper

2.5 ml/¹⁄₂ tsp gluten-free mustard powder

60 ml/4 tbsp sunflower or olive oil

30 ml/2 tbsp lemon juice

15 ml/1 tbsp white wine vinegar

250 ml/8 fl oz/1 cup dairy-free milk

1 Blend the flour, arrowroot, sugar, salt, pepper and mustard powder in a saucepan.

2 Stir in the oil, lemon juice and vinegar. When well blended, gradually stir in the milk.

3 Bring to the boil, stirring, and cook until thickened. Cover with a circle of wet greaseproof paper and leave to cool. Taste and re-season, if necessary. Turn into a clean, screw-topped jar and store in the fridge for up to 2 weeks.

Tolerant to ...	Variations
Dairy	Use cows' milk – full-cream for under-5s, semi-skimmed for older children.
Wheat	Use plain (all-purpose) flour instead of the potato flour and arrowroot.

No-allergen Hard Cheese

This makes a high-protein, low-fat cheese that tastes rather like Red Leicester. For the purposes of this book, I had to make it totally allergen-free but I think you get a better result if you make it with cashew nuts, so unless your child is allergic to tree nuts, I recommend you use the version given in the Variations. If you are planning to grate it, store it in the freezer and grate from frozen. If your child is allergic to citrus fruits, use white wine vinegar instead of lemon juice.

MAKES ABOUT 225 G/8 OZ

---

30 ml/2 tbsp powdered gelatine

30 ml/2 tbsp lemon juice

50 g/2 oz/¹/₂ cup potato flour

250 ml/8 fl oz/1 cup water or dairy-free milk 🥛

425 g/15 oz/1 large can of chick peas (garbanzos), thoroughly drained ☻

10 ml/2 tsp onion salt

1 small canned pimiento cap, drained

---

1 Sprinkle the gelatine over the lemon juice, stir and leave to soften.

2 Blend the flour with the water or milk in a saucepan. Bring to the boil, stirring all the time, until the mixture is thick and leaves the sides of the pan clean. Reduce the heat and cook for 3 minutes, stirring all the time.

3 Stir in the lump of softened gelatine and continue to stir until completely dissolved.

4 Put the chick peas in a blender or food processor with the onion salt and pimiento. Blend until smooth, stopping and scraping down the sides as necessary (this will take several minutes).

5 Add the flour mix and continue to run the machine until completely blended. Taste and add a little more lemon juice or salt to get a stronger flavour, if you prefer.

6 Line a 450 g/1 lb loaf tin (pan) with clingfilm (plastic wrap), leaving enough hanging over the sides of the tin to wrap completely. Tip the mixture into the tin and level the surface. Wrap the remaining clingfilm over the surface. Leave to cool, then chill until firm. Remove from the tin and wrap in another plastic bag. Store in the fridge or freezer.

Tolerant to ...	Variations
◉ Nuts	Use 100 g/4 oz/1 cup raw cashew nuts instead of the chick peas.

Apple and Date Spread

MAKES 1 POT

2 large eating (dessert) apples, peeled, cored and chopped

100 g/4 oz/²/₃ cup stoned (pitted) dates, chopped

2.5 ml/¹/₂ tsp ground cinnamon

175 ml/6 fl oz/³/₄ cup water

1 Put all the ingredients in a saucepan and cover with a lid. Bring to the boil, reduce the heat and simmer for 15 minutes until really soft.

2 Mash the cooked fruit with a potato masher, or purée in a blender or food processor. Cover and leave until completely cold. Transfer to a sealed container and store in the fridge.

Non-dairy Soft Cheese

MAKES ABOUT 100 G/4 OZ/¹/₂ CUP

250 ml/8 fl oz/1 cup plain sheep's yoghurt ☙

1 Line a sieve (strainer) with a new disposable kitchen cloth. Place it over a bowl.

2 Tip the yoghurt into the sieve and fold the edges of the cloth over so they don't drip. Place in the fridge for several hours or, preferably, overnight.

3 The whey will drip through into the bowl, leaving a soft, white cheese in the sieve. Store the cheese in an airtight container in the fridge for up to a week.

Tolerant to ...	Variations
☙ Soya	Use soya yoghurt.

Non-dairy Soft Cheese with Chives: Add 15 ml/1 tbsp of snipped fresh chives to the cheese and flavour it with salt and pepper to taste.

Non-dairy Soft Cheese with Garlic and Herbs: Add a small crushed garlic clove and 5 ml/1 tsp of dried mixed herbs to the cheese.

Whipped Rice Cream

This makes a good dairy-free substitute for double cream.

MAKES 250 ML/8 FL OZ/1 CUP

100 g/4 oz/½ cup dairy-free margarine

120 ml/4 fl oz/½ cup rice milk

7.5 ml/1½ tsp arrowroot

1 Melt the margarine in a saucepan. Add the milk and whisk in the arrowroot.

2 Bring to the boil, stirring, until slightly thickened. Leave to cool, then chill.

3 Whisk with an electric whisk until thick, then chill again until required. It will keep for a week or two in the fridge.

Whipped Dream Cream

This makes another good substitute for whipped cream, but it is only suitable if your child can tolerate soya. If not, use the Whipped Rice Cream recipe on page 181. Soya Dream, a cream substitute, is widely available in supermarkets.

MAKES ABOUT 300 ML/½ PT/1¼ CUPS

5 ml/1 tsp powdered gelatine

15 ml/1 tbsp water

150 ml/¼ pt/⅔ cup Soya Dream, chilled

A little caster (superfine) sugar (optional)

1 Put the gelatine in a small bowl and add the water. Leave to soften for 5 minutes, then stand the bowl in a pan of simmering water and stir until the gelatine has completely dissolved.

2 Pour the Soya Dream into a bowl and whisk with an electric or hand whisk until thick and almost doubled in bulk. Whisk in the gelatine and sweeten to taste, if liked.

3 Chill in the fridge for at least 30 minutes to set.

Nut Milk

This is a delicious alternative to soya, goats' or sheep's milk but is only suitable if your child can tolerate nuts. It is particularly nice on cereal and for making pancakes etc. It is good to drink too – especially when chilled. You must use plain, raw nuts, not roasted ones.

MAKES ABOUT 600 ML/1 PT/2½ CUPS

175 g/6 oz/1½ cups chopped mixed nuts

750 ml/1¼ pts/3 cups water

1   Put the nuts and half the water in a blender or food processor. Run the machine until the mixture is as smooth as possible. Add the remaining water and blend briefly again.

2   Strain the mixture through a sieve (strainer), lined with a new disposable kitchen cloth, into a bowl.

3   Gather up the corners of the cloth and squeeze it well to extract the last of the liquid. Store in a clean screw-topped bottle in the fridge.

Nut Cream

This makes a great alternative to dairy cream but is only suitable if your child can tolerate nuts.

SERVES 4

50 g/2 oz/½ cup ground almonds or hazelnuts (filberts)

60 ml/4 tbsp cold water

10 ml/2 tsp caster (superfine) sugar

1   Blend the nuts with the water.

2   Stir in the sugar. The mixture should be a soft, dropping consistency. Use as required.

Cornmeal Custard

This makes lovely yellow custard. If your child can't tolerate corn, use double the quantity of rice flour instead and add a few drops of yellow food colouring to the sauce.

SERVES 4

---

15 g/¹/₂ oz/2 tbsp cornmeal

30 ml/2 tbsp granulated sugar

450 ml/³/₄ pt/2 cups dairy-free milk 🥛

2.5 ml/¹/₂ tsp natural vanilla essence (extract)

15 g/¹/₂ oz/1 tbsp dairy-free margarine 🥛

---

1 Mix the cornmeal and sugar together in a bowl. Make into a smooth paste with a little of the milk.

2 Bring the remaining milk to the boil in a saucepan. Pour on to the corn paste, stirring all the time, then add the vanilla essence.

3 Return to the saucepan and bring to the boil, stirring all the time. Cook fairly rapidly for 5 minutes, stirring. Whisk in the margarine until thoroughly blended. Serve hot.

Tolerant to ...	Variations
🥛 Dairy	Use cows' milk – full-cream for under-5s, semi-skimmed for older children – and butter or ordinary margarine.

Wheat-free/Gluten-free Play Dough

The quantity of salt will remind your children that this is not for eating!

MAKES ABOUT 350 G/12 OZ

225 g/8 oz/2 cups rice flour

225 g/8 oz/2 cups salt

15 ml/1 tbsp cream of tartar

30 ml/2 tbsp sunflower oil

250 ml/8 fl oz/1 cup water

A few drops of food colouring (optional)

1 Mix the flour, salt and cream of tartar in a saucepan.

2 Add the oil and gradually blend in the water and food colouring, if using.

3 Cook over a moderate heat, stirring, until the mixture is stiff and leaves the sides of the pan clean.

4 Leave until cool enough to handle, then knead gently on the work surface until smooth. Store in an airtight container.

USEFUL ADDRESSES

Action Against Allergy
7 Strawberry Hill Road
Twickenham
TW1 4QQ
Tel: 020 8892 2711
www.actionagainstallergy.co.uk

Allergy UK
(The operational name of the British Allergy Foundation)
Deepdene House
30 Bellgrove Road
Welling
Kent DA16 3PY
Tel: 020 8303 8525
Helpline: 020 8303 8583
www.allergyuk.org

Anaphylaxis Campaign
Tel: 01252 542029
www.anaphylaxis.org.uk

Coeliac UK
PO Box 220
High Wycombe
Bucks HP11 2HY
Tel: 01494 437278
www.coeliac.co.uk

ggfi
www.ggfi.co.uk
(Specialist foods, including guar gum)

Goodness Direct (online only)
www.GoodnessDirect.co.uk
(Information, nutritional advice including baby weaning)

Lifestyle Healthcare Ltd
Tel: 01491 570000
www.glutenfree.co.uk
(Specialist foods by mail order)

INDEX